STIR FRY COOKBOOK

2nd Edition

55 Stir Fry Recipes That Are Healthy, Tasty & Easy to Make!

Olivia Rogers

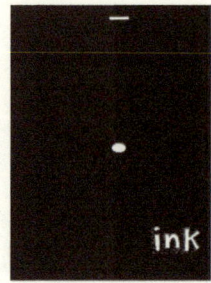

First published in 2019 by Venture Ink Publishing

Copyright © The Menu At Home 2019

All rights reserved.

No part of this book may be reproduced in any form without permission in writing from the author. No part of this publication may be reproduced or transmitted in any form or by any means, mechanic, electronic, photocopying, recording, by any storage or retrieval system, or transmitted by email without the permission in writing from the author and publisher.

Requests to the publisher for permission should be addressed to publishing@ventureink.co

For more information about the contents of this book or questions to the author, please contact Olivia Rogers at olivia@themenuathome.com

Disclaimer

This book provides wellness management information in an informative and educational manner only, with information that is general in nature and that is not specific to you, the reader. The contents of this book are intended to assist you and other readers in your personal wellness efforts. Consult your physician regarding the applicability of any information provided in this book to you.

Nothing in this book should be construed as personal advice or diagnosis, and must not be used in this manner. The information provided about conditions is general in nature. This information does not cover all possible uses, actions, precautions, side-effects, or interactions of medicines, or medical procedures. The information in this book should not be considered as complete and does not cover all diseases, ailments, physical conditions, or their treatment.

You should consult with your physician before beginning any exercise, weight loss, or health care program. This book should not be used in place of a call or visit to a competent health-care professional. You should consult a health care professional before adopting any of the suggestions in this book or before drawing inferences from it.

Any decision regarding treatment and medication for your condition should be made with the advice and consultation of a qualified health care professional. If you have, or suspect you have, a health-care problem, then you should immediately contact a qualified health care professional for treatment.

No Warranties: The author and publisher don't guarantee or warrant the quality, accuracy, completeness, timeliness, appropriateness or suitability of the information in this book, or of any product or services referenced in this book.

The information in this book is provided on an "as is" basis and the author and publisher make no representations or warranties of any kind with respect to this information. This book may contain inaccuracies, typographical errors, or other errors.

Liability Disclaimer: The publisher, author, and other parties involved in the creation, production, provision of information, or delivery of this book specifically disclaim any responsibility, and shall not be held liable for any damages, claims, injuries, losses, liabilities, costs, or obligations including any direct, indirect, special, incidental, or consequences damages (collectively known as "Damages") whatsoever and howsoever caused, arising out of, or in connection with the use or misuse of the site and the information contained within it, whether such Damages arise in contract, tort, negligence, equity, statute law, or by way of other legal theory.

Table of Contents

Disclaimer	3
Who is this book for?	7
What will this book teach you?	9
Introduction	11
Selecting the Equipment	13
Chapter 1: Pork Stir-Fry Recipes	15
Chapter 2: Poultry Stir-Fry Recipes	43
Chapter 3: Stir-Fry Beef Recipes	77
Chapter 4: Marine Stir-Fry Recipes	105
Chapter 5: Vegetables Stir-Fry Recipes	135
Conclusion	161
Final Words	163

Who is this book for?

Do you want to learn the art of stir-frying with quick recipes for you, family and friends? In this book, I have included recipes that will demand 20-40 minutes of your time.

Others will need an hour cooking time or preparing some of the ingredients in advance before proceeding with the method. They are there to give you an idea of what your friends and family can enjoy during a weekend or dinner visit.

In general, making stir fries doesn't need too much time. Here, you have recipes that will feed the entire family, if it not a meal for two.

It gets interesting as you prepare using the step-by-step method I have used to explain the process of making every meal in this book.

By reading this book, you will be satisfying the urge of familiarizing yourself with the stir-frying cuisines. We all know how cuisines from China, Japan, and Thailand are mouthwatering. The good news is that they are available in this book, and customized for you to give a shot!

So, if getting some tasty stir-fried meals is in your line of duty, then take your time, read this book and thank me later!

What will this book teach you?

This book will teach you on the following:

55 detailed stir-fry recipes that take a considerable amount of time. I have divided them into five chapters: Pork, Chicken, Beef, Marine and Vegetable stir-fries.

Explanation of different terms used in stir fry recipes. You will be able to understand what you are venturing in before using the wok.

Images of every recipe to give you an idea of what the entire plate will look like when you serve.

Introduction

Many chefs and moms all over the globe are embracing the art of stir-frying to create a dishy meal for the family or consumers in general.

In the course of cooking, you will learn that this cooking technique involves cutting down of food into small pieces before cooking them rapidly with excess heat and little oil.

The sequence of adding to the wok/pan considers putting first what will take longer to prepare and the ingredients needing shorter following later.

When the instructions direct you to cut down into small pieces, it means that you are providing a perfect venue for tenderizing, either wholly or relatively depending on how large or small the pieces.

You are required to prepare the ingredients by removing the unnecessary as per the directions to achieve the best results.

All food requirements in this book can join the wok after proper cutting, dicing and stripping.

In all recipes, one of the instructions is to burn the oil until it is smoking hot. At such high temperatures, the fat begins to break down.

So, your oil selection should be able withstand high amounts of heat. Vegetable oil is an excellent choice, but peanut is the best since it has a high smoking point, not to mention the flavor.

There will be liquids that you will need to be aware of in the course of reading the book. Soy sauce, hot and sweet chili, sherry wine (fortified type) and various kinds of broths.

For the soups, you should know how to prepare them. Most of the sauces should be thick, so the ingredients you choose are a significant factor to the overall effect on flavor.

Selecting the Equipment

You will need the following when preparing stir-fries:

- A wok, large skillet or a large non-stick frying pan. If you own them all, that's great.

- Spatula or chopsticks

- Bowls of different sizes

- Serving platters

- Colander – a bowl-shaped strainer

- Paper/kitchen towels

- Chopping board and knives

- Spoons and forks

- Blender/food processor

You can add other items if required while stir-frying. I have specified other things you might need in individual recipes apart from the usual ones. You can mark them as you continue reading.

Chapter 1

Pork Stir-Fry Recipes

Most of us have consumed pork for a long time. However, stir-frying it changes every other view you might have about this type of meat. Check this collection of recipes to make the best out of pork.

1. Ginger-Lemon Pork

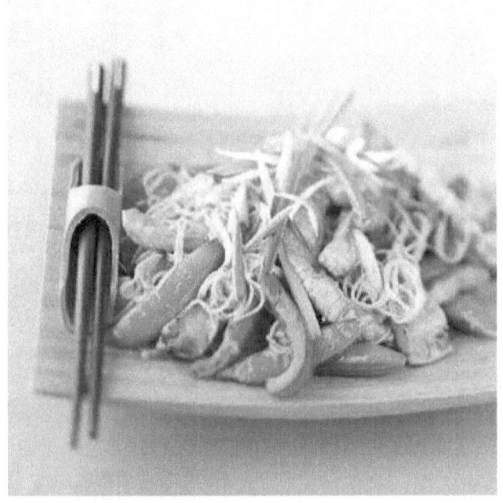

Cooking time: 30 minutes
Serving: 4

Ingredients

- Pork tenderloin – 1 pound
- Angel hair pasta – 8 ounces
- Vegetable oil – 1

- Cornstarch – 1 tablespoon
- Pepper – 1/8 teaspoon
- Salt – ¼ teaspoon
- Sugar-snap peas – 6 ounces
- Fresh lemon juice – ½ cup
- Sweet red pepper, cut it into ¼-inch broad slices – 1
- Fresh grated ginger – 1 teaspoon
- Bottled chili sauce – 2 tablespoons
- Grated lemon rind – 1 teaspoon
- Chopped scallions – ¼ cup

Directions

1. Start by cooking the angel hair pasta following directions on the package. Drain when ready and rinse with cold water. After rinsing, put it aside and move to the next step. Use a meat board and knife to cut the pork tenderloin into ¼-inch thick slices.

2. With all ingredients measured, mix the pork with cornstarch, vegetable oil, salt, and pepper in a large bowl. Trim the sugar-snap peas and then proceed to heat the oil (1 tablespoon) in a skillet on extreme heat.

3. Put the sliced pork in the skillet and stir-fry for three minutes until it browns. Add the peas and pepper strips. After stir-frying for another three minutes, empty the contents in a large bowl.

4. Back to the skillet, boil sugar and a quarter of the lemon juice for three minutes until they turn caramel (yellow-

brown). Add the remaining ¼ cup of lemon juice, chili sauce, ground lemon rind, and ginger.

5. Stir a bit and then add the vegetables, pork, and pasta. Cook by stirring so that everything heats through. Switch off the heat and sprinkle with scallions after serving.

2. Spicy Black Bean Sauce Pork

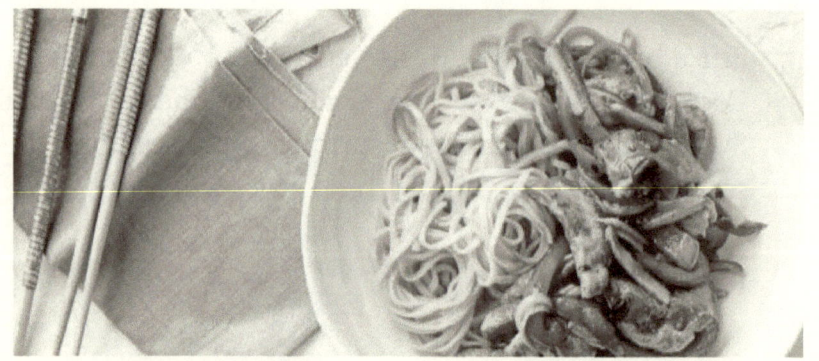

Cooking time: 20 minutes
Serving: 2

Ingredients

- Pork tenderloin, trim and cut into strips – 300 grams
- Frying oil
- Corn flour – 1 tablespoon
- Sliced green pepper – 1
- Sliced onion – 1
- Shredded Ginger– 1
- Chili flakes – 1 pinch
- Crushed Sichuan peppercorns – 1 tablespoon
- Black bean sauce – 6 tablespoons
- Cooked egg noodles. Heat before serving.

Directions

1. Here, you need to season the pork first by tossing with corn flour. After that, take a wok and heat two

tablespoons of oil until hot. Put the coated pork in the wok and stir-fry until golden.

2. Put the pork in a bowl and proceed to add one more tablespoon of oil in the wok followed by the cut onions and pepper.

3. Stir-fry to soften the pepper and onions. Add ginger, chili, and peppercorns and cook them for one minute.

4. Put the black bean sauce and add water (100ml). Reduce the heat to medium for the food to simmer.

5. Put the pork back to the wok and toss it until it is heated through. Switch off the heat and serve together with noodles.

3. Sticky Pork and Mange Tout

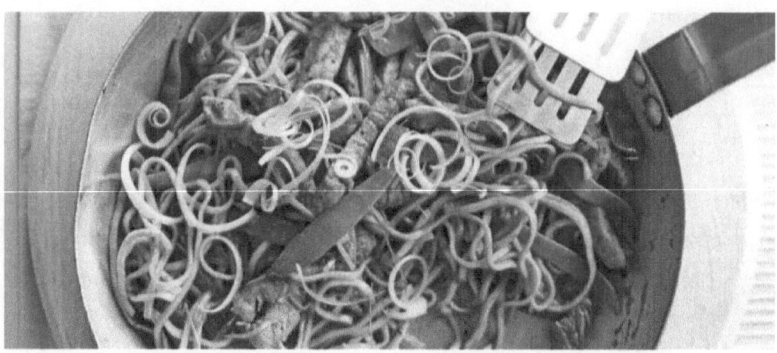

Cooking time: 20 minutes
Serving: 2

Ingredients

- Thin pork slices, cut into strips – 300 grams
- Corn flour – 1 tablespoon
- Egg noodles, dried – 100 grams
- Frying oil
- Mangetout, halved – 100 grams
- Honey – 1 tablespoon
- Lemon, juiced – 1
- Chili sauce – 2 tablespoons
- Soy sauce – 2 tablespoons

Directions

1. Cook the noodles in a pot following the package instructions and make sure they are well drained. As

the noodles cook, prepare the pork by tossing it with corn flour.

2. When the pork is ready, take a wok or a big non-stick fry pan and heat one tablespoon of oil. Put the meat in the wok or pan and stir-fry it for two minutes before you scoop it out and set aside.

3. Add mangetout and some of the spring onions and then toss for some minutes. Put the pork back and add lemon, soy, honey, and chili.

4. Splash in some water and let the food bubble for at least 3 minutes or until you get a sauce.

5. Finish up by tossing in the noodles until they are heated through. Sprinkle the remaining spring onions before serving.

4. Pork with Lo Mein Noodles and Vegetables

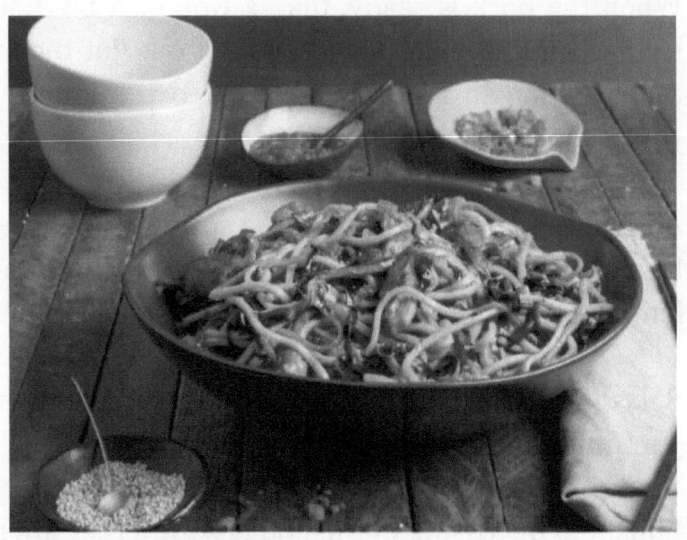

Cooking time: 40 minutes
Serving 4

Ingredients

- Fresh Lo Mein noodles – 450 grams
- Kosher salt
- Boneless country-style pork ribs – 450 grams
- Sugar – 3 tablespoons
- Baking soda – 1 teaspoon
- Oyster sauce – 3 tablespoons
- Soy sauce – 3 tablespoons
- Balsamic vinegar – 2 tablespoons
- Dry sherry – 2 tablespoons
- Toasted sesame oil – 1 tablespoon

- Fish sauce – 1 tablespoon
- Neutral oil such as canola or peanut – 3 tablespoons, divided
- Ginger knob, minced – 1
- Cornstarch – 1 tablespoon
- Minced medium garlic cloves – 3
- Shredded and cored purple cabbage – 1 ½ cups (150 grams)
- Scallions, green parts thinly sliced, cut the white parts into 1-inch pieces – 4
- Cored Napa cabbage, or shredded Chinese broccoli – 1 ½ cups (150 grams)
- Carrots, cut into long thin strips – 1 cup (75 grams)

Directions

1. Cook the noodles using salted boiling water according to the instructions. Make sure they are firm to be eaten and separated before draining and setting aside. Trim the pork to get rid of excess fat before you cut it into 2 inches long and a ¼-inch wide slices.

2. Put baking soda in a bowl and stir after adding half a cup of cold water. Put the pork in the bowl with the baking soda mixture and stir to get a full coating. In that state, let them stay for the next 15 minutes.

3. As you wait, take another medium bowl and whisk together the following: sugar, oyster sauce, soy sauce, sesame oil, vinegar, fish sauce, wine, and cornstarch. When the sugar is fully dissolved, set it aside.

4. Drain the pork and rinse it with water (cold) before using paper towels to pat dry. Rinse and dry the bowl that had pork and add the meat back. Add two tablespoons of the sauce you prepared in step 5 and mix thoroughly.

5. Take a wok or a skillet and heat a tablespoon of neutral oil on medium heat until it shimmers. Proceed by adding garlic, ginger and the white scallion parts and stir-fry them for 30 seconds.

6. Switch the heat to high and then add the cabbage, carrots and Napa cabbage or broccoli depending on what you chose. Stir and toss until the contents you added in step 10 are cooked through. Are they ready? Transfer everything to a plate.

7. Clean the skillet or wok by wiping out. After cleaning, put one tablespoon of neutral oil and heat until it's smoking hot. Add noodles to the wok and toss as you stir until they become hot.

8. Now, add the earlier made pork together with the rest of the sauce, veggies, and noodles. Stir-fry everything so that the meat can mix with the added ingredients.

9. Put the meat and lo Mein on a platter and sprinkle the green scallion parts. If you still got the sesame seeds, sprinkle along. Serve right away.

5. Spicy Ground Pork with Cucumbers

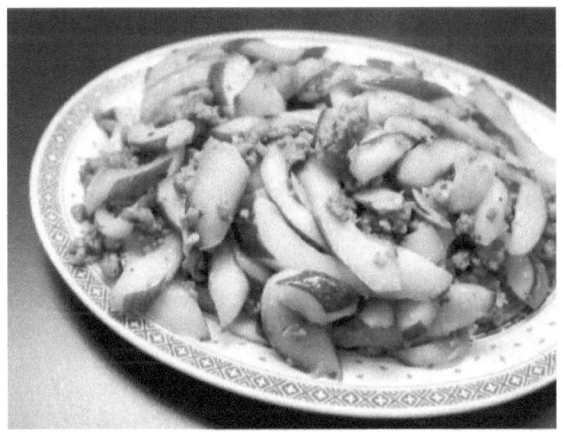

Cooking time: 1 hour
Serving: 2-4

Ingredients

Marinated pork ingredients

- Ground pork – 225 grams
- Shaoxing wine (traditional Chinese wine made from rice) – 1 teaspoon
- Soy sauce – 1 teaspoon
- Asian fish sauce – 1 teaspoon
- Vegetable oil – 1 teaspoon
- Cornstarch – ½ teaspoon

Sauce and stir-fry ingredients

- Soy sauce – 1 teaspoon
- Cornstarch – ½ teaspoon

- Toasted sesame oil – 1 teaspoon
- Chili flakes for the taste – 1 teaspoon
- Vegetable oil – 1 teaspoon and 1 tablespoon, divided
- Peeled and sliced garlic head – ½ head
- Cooked white rice and ready to serve

Other ingredients

- Large cucumbers - 2 pounds or 3
- Kosher salt – 1 ½ teaspoons

Directions

1. First, partially peel the cucumbers vertically in an alternating peeling and un-peeling manner. Extract the seeds before you cut them into ¼-inch slices. Put the cucumbers in a bowl and add some salt. Toss and mix so that the cucumbers can release some water. It will take you a minute or so. Let it stay in that condition for 30 minutes.

2. As you wait for the cucumbers, it is now time to marinate the pork. Take a small bowl and put the ground pork. Follow by adding the following to the meat: soy sauce, oil, Shaoxing wine, cornstarch and fish sauce. Mix everything thoroughly and refrigerate for 30 minutes or so. Do you have time? Let it stay overnight. A good idea is to prepare it before practicing this recipe.

3. In the meantime, take a small bowl and add the following: water, sesame oil, soy sauce and cornstarch. Mix them thoroughly before setting the bowl aside. Go

back to the cucumbers and drain them before rinsing with running cold water. Drain them again and pat dry using paper towels.

4. With all the above ready, take a wok and heat a teaspoon of vegetable oil over high heat until it's hot. Put the marinated pork and spread it out using a spatula to get a thin layer in the wok. Let it cook for 30 seconds and don't disturb it as you wait.

5. After 30 seconds are over, split the pork into smaller pieces using the spatula. Add the chili flakes and stir-fry until the pork turns golden brown. Put the contents in a bowl and set them aside.

6. Clean the wok by wiping. After that, add a teaspoon of vegetable oil and overheat. When the oil is hot, add garlic and stir for the next 10 seconds before adding the cucumbers. Continue to mix for at least two minutes.

7. Put the pork back and keep stirring. When the pork has mixed well with the already put ingredients, take the sauce and mix a little with a spoon before pouring it to the wok.

8. After the pour, cook and stir until the cucumbers become glossy. It will take you about 30 seconds. Switch off the heat and empty the wok to a plate. Serve the stir-fry immediately with the cooked rice.

6. Sweet and Sour Pork

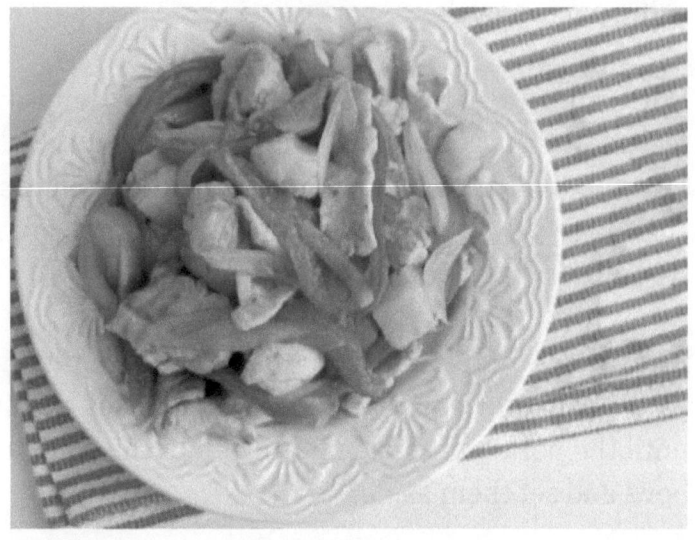

Note: Water-velveting makes the meat strips tender. Prepare this recipe if you have time, probably on the weekend if not during the night.

Cooking time: 1hour
Serving: 2

Ingredients

Pork Ingredients

- Cornstarch – 2 teaspoons
- A lightly beaten egg white – 1 tablespoon
- Chinese rice wine (Shaoxing wine) – 2 teaspoons
- Pork loin, 1/8-inch slices – ½ pound (225 grams)
- Kosher salt – ¼ teaspoon

- Vegetable or canola oil – 1 teaspoon
- Water – 6 cups

Stir-fry ingredients

- Tomato paste – 1 teaspoon
- Canned pineapple chunks – ½ cup
- Canned pineapple juice – 4 tablespoons
- Soy sauce – 2 teaspoons
- Rice vinegar – 2 tablespoons
- Cornstarch – 1 teaspoon
- Sesame oil – ½ teaspoon
- Vegetable or canola oil – 1 tablespoon
- Red bell pepper, seed and stem it before slicing into ½-inch thick lengthwise slices – ½
- Green bell pepper prepared the same way as the red one – ½
- Small white onion, cut into ½-inch thick slices – ½
- Cooked white rice

Directions

Preparing the pork

1. Take a small bowl and thoroughly mix the cornstarch, egg white, rice wine, and salt. Get another bowl and put the pork in. Pour the mixture you prepared in step 1 over the meat and toss it for the best coating results. Let it refrigerate for about 30 minutes.

2. After the ½ hour wait, put water in a wok and boil it using high heat. At boiling point, add oil. Add the coated pork in the wok and stir using chopsticks (a strainer comes in handy too), to separate the pieces. Continue cooking for the next 40 seconds, until the pork turns opaque or nearly cooked through.

3. Drain the contents using a bowl-shaped strainer and shake after each fetch to make sure most of the water gets out. When the wok is empty, wipe and dry it thoroughly.

Preparing the stir-fry

1. Take a small bowl and mix the following: Tomato paste, pineapple juice, soy sauce, rice vinegar, cornstarch and sesame oil. Go back to the wok and heat vegetable or canola oil until it's smoking hot. Add both green and red bell peppers, then stir-fry for the next 30 seconds.

2. Add the pork and keep stir-frying until you see some brown spots which will take at least 2 minutes. Get a spatula and move the pork and veggies to the sides of the wok. Add sauce at the center spot you made after moving the meat and vegetables.

3. Let the sauce boil as you slightly stir then start tossing the pork and vegetables for the sauce to coat everything. After an even coat, stop heating and toss in the pineapple chunks. Serve the stir-fried food immediately with the cooked rice.

7. Pork with Kale and Spring Onions

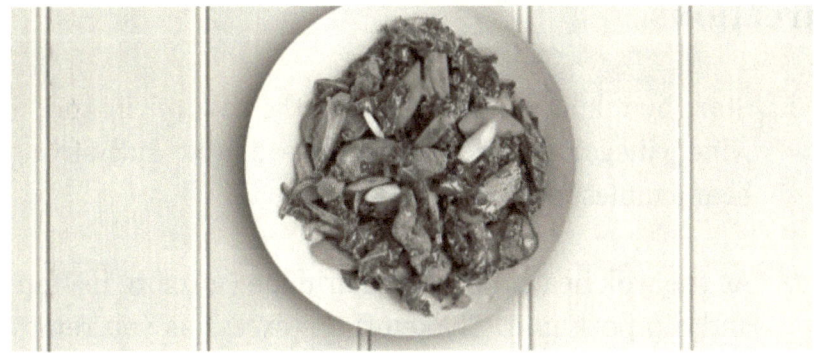

Here is a great supper option if you want to have a taste of some sweet pork with chili. Ginger and mirin (Japanese rice wine) takes this recipe to another level. You can choose to serve with rice or noodles.

Cooking time: 20 minutes
Serving: 4

Ingredients

- Rice wine vinegar – 1 tablespoon
- Soy sauce – 1 tablespoon
- Mirin – 2 tablespoons
- Trimmed pork tenderloin, cut into strips – 1 pound
- Groundnut oil
- Seeded and finely chopped red chili – 1
- Grated ginger – thumb size
- Crushed garlic clove – 1
- Carrots, peeled and thinly sliced – 2
- Kales, wash and chop them – 200 grams

- Diced spring onions – 3

Directions

1. Start by taking a bowl and mix the soy, mirin and rice wine vinegar. After mixing, take a wok and strongly heat a tablespoon of oil.

2. As the wok heats, take the marinade (mixture in step 1) and dip pork in it. Shake off the excess as you remove, and put the meat in a bowl. Follow by frying in batches until you see a golden color.

3. When golden, take the meat out of the wok and wipe it clean. Heat another tablespoon of oil until it's hot. Follow by frying the garlic, chili, and ginger until the smell reaches you.

4. At fragrance, add carrots then stir-fry for two minutes. Add the onions, kales, marinade and the pork, in that order.

5. Let it cook for 7-8 minutes so that the pork cooks through. When the meat is ready, serve with rice or noodles.

8. Caramelized Pork – Vietnamese

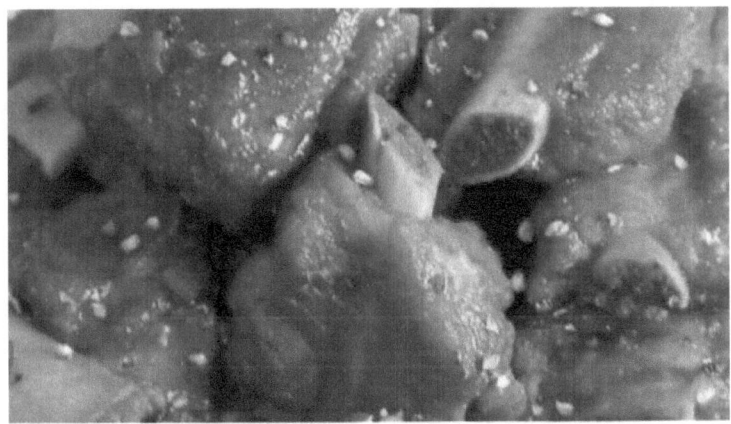

If you cook ordinary or jasmine rice, here is a quick recipe to serve with it.

Cooking time: 35 minutes
Serving: 4

Ingredients

- White sugar – 1 cup
- Vegetable oil – 1 tablespoon
- Pork spare ribs, sliced into 1-inch pieces – 2 pounds
- Chopped green chili pepper – 1
- Green onions, sliced into 2-inch lengths – 2
- Ground black pepper – 1 teaspoon
- Finely chopped shallots (bulb onions) – 2
- Minced garlic cloves – 2
- Salt
- Thinly sliced green onion, separated into rings – 1 tablespoon

- Sesame oil – 1 teaspoon

Directions

1. Strongly heat the wok or a heavy skillet. When it's smoking hot, add oil in a drizzling manner. After the oil, pour sugar on it. Proceed to continuously stir the mixture until the sugar dissolves and turns to light brown.

2. What you just did is caramelizing the sugar (turning into a caramel color). Now, put the pork, some of the green onions, chili and black pepper, shallots, garlic cloves, and salt.

3. Toss the meat together with the added ingredients until the pork turns golden brown. Take sesame oil and drizzle it over the pork and veggies. Turn the heat to low so that the food can simmer.

4. When the juices are almost absorbed, put the heat back to high and stir the food until the sauce thickens and coats the pork. It should take you 5 minutes.

5. Use a tablespoon to sprinkle the remaining green onions over the pork and vegetables before serving.

9. Spicy Pork

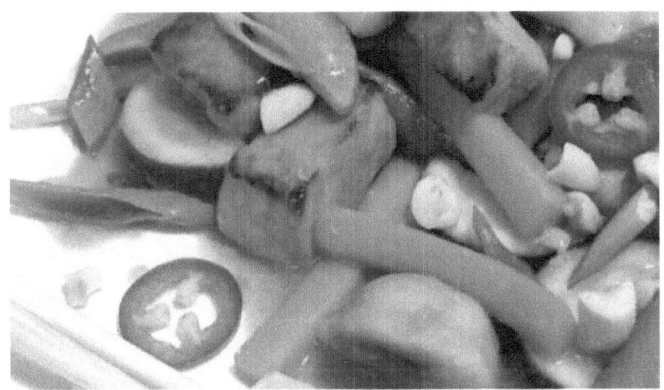

This recipe is way too spicy so make sure you have lots of white rice to cover for that.

Cooking time: 1 hour
Serving: 4

Ingredients

- Cornstarch – 1 tablespoon and 1 teaspoon, separate
- Soy sauce – 2 tablespoons and 1 tablespoon, separate
- Cubed pork tenderloin – 1 pound
- Squeezed lime – 1
- Rice vinegar – 2 tablespoons
- Dark sesame oil – 3 tablespoons
- Fresh and minced ginger root – 3 teaspoons
- Peanut oil – 1 tablespoon
- Carrots, cut into long thin strips – ½ cup
- Chopped green chili peppers – 2
- Sugar snap peas, cut into long strips – ½ cup

- Green onions, chopped – ¼ cup
- Chili oil – 2 teaspoons
- Finely chopped peanuts – ¼ cup

Directions

1. Get a medium bowl and put the following in it: soy sauce (two tablespoons) cornstarch (one tablespoon) and water. Mix them thoroughly to get a smooth texture. Stir the pork cubes in the mixture you just prepared. Cover the bowl and refrigerate the marinated pork for at least 30 minutes.

2. Meanwhile, take a small bowl and mix lime, soy sauce (1 tablespoon) cornstarch (1 teaspoon) and sesame oil. Mix them before setting them aside for later use. After 30 minutes in the refrigerator, remove the pork.

3. Turn on the heat, place a wok or large skillet with peanut oil in it until it becomes hot. Stir in the ginger, chili pepper, and salt for a minute.

4. Put the marinated pork in the wok together with marinade and sugar snap peas. Stir-fry for the next 6-8 minutes for the pork to tenderize.

5. When the meat is tenderized, put the lime mixture. Lower the heat to medium for the sauce to simmer and thicken. It should take you another 6-8 minutes. Switch off the heat and stir in chili oil, peanuts, and green onions before serving.

10. Pork and Pepper

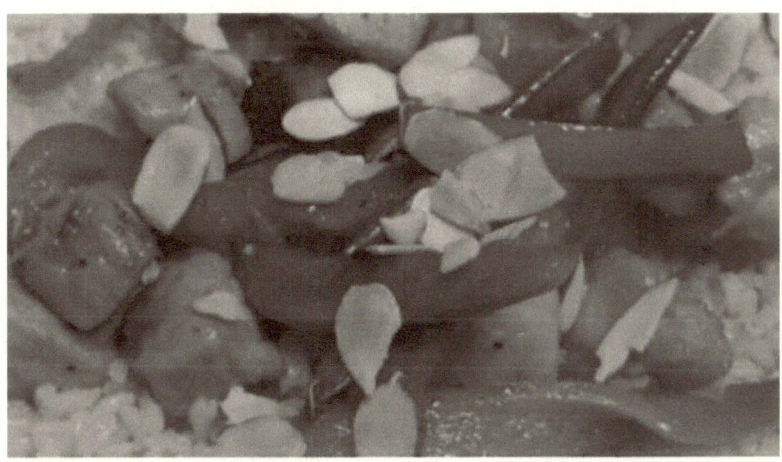

You can substitute the pork with beef or chicken if pork is not a favorite when combined with pepper. You can also prepare the marinade or choose not to. In short, you can bend the rules here.

Cooking time: 1 hour 10 minutes
Serving: 4

Ingredients

Marinade ingredients

- Garlic, minced – 2 tablespoons
- Rice wine vinegar – ¼ cup
- Olive oil – 5 tablespoons
- Brown sugar – 1 tablespoon
- Salt and pepper

Stir-fry ingredients

- Boneless pork meat, cut into small bite-size pieces – 4 pounds
- Fresh ginger root, finely chopped – 3 tablespoons
- Vegetable oil – 5 tablespoons
- Hot chili paste – 1 tablespoon
- Green, red, and yellow bell peppers, cut into strips – 1 each
- Teriyaki sauce (homemade for taste preference) – 5 tablespoons
- Fresh mint, chopped – 2 tablespoons
- Briefly cooked splintered almonds – ¼ cup
- Salt and pepper

Directions

1. Get a large bowl and mix the following: garlic, rice wine vinegar, olive oil, brown sugar, salt, and pepper. When the mixture is ready, stir the pork in and leave it for 30 minutes, at room temperature. After the ½ hour wait, heat a wok or a large frying pan using medium heat. Do not add oil.

2. When heated, put the almonds in the dry wok and toast to get a golden-brown color and a sweet aroma. After cooking, place them on a platter or bowl and set them aside.

3. Back in the wok, heat the vegetable oil over medium to high heat. Put the marinated pork, chili paste, and

ginger and stir as the pork fries. The rest of the marinade is not useful after this.

4. Put the teriyaki sauce in the wok or pan and increase the heat. With the heat at high level, stir and cook until the pork goes white.

5. Now, it is time to stir the peppers in as you continue to stir until almost all liquid is gone. After, add the almond slivers you toasted together with mint in the frying food. Switch off the heat when the food is ready and serve.

11. Pork, Ginger, and Apple with Hoisin Sauce

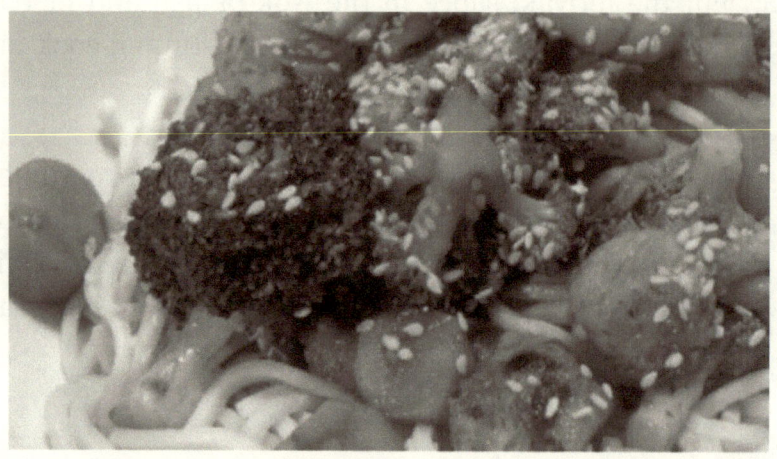

Cooking time: 40 minutes
Serving: 3

Ingredients

- Brown sugar – 2 tablespoons
- Hoisin sauce – 2 tablespoons
- Soy sauce – 6 tablespoons
- Pork loin, cut into strips – 1 pound
- Applesauce – ½ cup
- Cornstarch – 1 ½ tablespoons
- Sesame oil – ½ teaspoon
- Peanut oil – 2 tablespoons
- Broccoli florets – 3 cups
- Fresh ginger root, chopped – 1 tablespoon

Directions

1. In a small bowl, put brown sugar, hoisin sauce, applesauce and soy sauce and whisk thoroughly to mix. Set the bowl aside once the mixture is even.

2. In another bowl, mix pork with cornstarch. Make sure the meat gets an even coat before setting it aside too. Take a wok or a large skillet and put sesame and peanut oils. Use medium to high heat for the temperature.

3. Put the pork in three batches in the heated oil. Now, cook until the pink color in the middle of meat pieces disappears. One batch should take you 2-3 minutes before putting the next.

4. After a nearly cooked gesture, put the pork in a plate aligned with paper towels to drain the oil. Back to the wok/skillet, without wiping, put ginger and stir for the next 30 seconds.

5. After stirring, add broccoli and stir until it's tender. Return the meat in the wok and pour the sauce mixture. Toss everything to get a good coating on the meat and broccoli. Is it ready? Serve while it's still hot.

42

Chapter 2

Poultry Stir-Fry Recipes

Most, if not all of the recipes in this section are perfect for a busy week. Tossing chicken for your family twice per week gets the meal ready before you even know it.

Most of the time, you will be using chicken breasts or thighs. Make sure your pieces are uniform when cutting and marinate when necessary. Also let the food cook before heading to the dining table for health reasons of course. Raw or undercooked meat can bring all the unwanted complications.

12. Szechuan/Sichuan Chicken

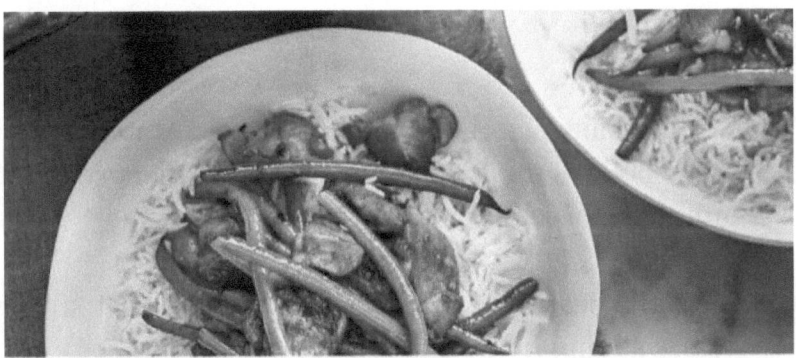

We start with a chicken stir-fry that is great for a midweek meal. The calories are also low if you like it that way.

Cooking time: 20 minutes
Serving: 2

Ingredients

- Frying oil – 2 tablespoons
- Trimmed green beans – 150 grams
- Thigh fillets from chicken, skinless and cut into chunks – 4 pieces
- Crushed Szechuan peppercorns – ¼ teaspoon
- Crushed garlic cloves – 2
- Dried chili flakes – 1 pinch
- Soy sauce – 1 tablespoon
- Grated ginger – 3cm chunk
- Honey – 2 teaspoons
- Sesame oil – ½ teaspoon
- Chinese rice wine (Shaoxing) – 1 tablespoon
- Rice or noodles, cooked to serve

Directions

1. Get a frying pan and put some salted water. Let the water boil before putting the beans. Let them cook for a minute before draining and setting them aside.

2. After the beans are ready, get a wok and heat strongly before adding frying oil.

3. Add the chicken pieces together with a pinch of salt (measure as preferred) and stir-fry for around 8 minutes until they turn golden and almost cooked.

4. Put the Szechuan peppercorns, green beans, and chili flakes. Let them cook together with the meat pieces for some minutes before adding ginger and garlic.

5. Continue cooking and stirring for 2 minutes. Add the remaining ingredients and toss to get a nice mixture. When ready, serve the chicken with whatever you have (noodles or rice).

13. Ginger Chicken

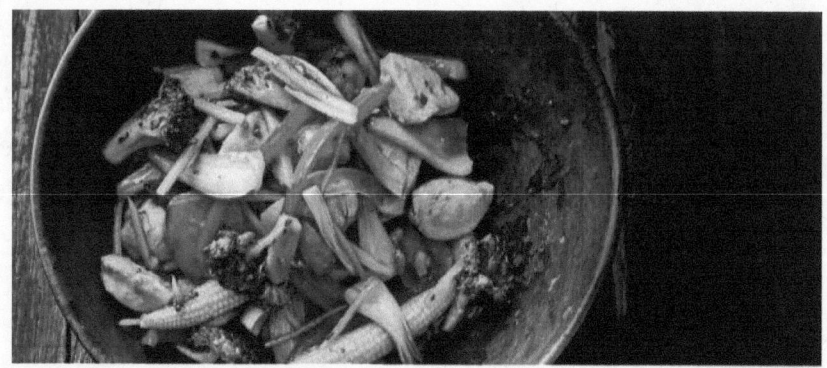

This recipe is also low in calories and simple to stir-fry. You get a packed sense of flavor in not more than 20 minutes.

Cooking time: 25 minutes
Serving 2

Ingredients

- Briefly cooked almonds – 30 grams
- Frying oil – 1 tablespoon
- Broccoli, cut into florets – ½ head (small)
- Chicken breasts, cut into small pieces – 2
- Thinly sliced or grated carrot – ½ teaspoon
- Baby corn – 100 grams
- Ginger, thumb-size, cut into small sticks – 2
- Baby Pak choy (Chinese white cabbage), cut into halves – 2
- Red pepper, sliced – ½
- Spring onions, 5cm slices – 2

Sauce ingredients

- Soy sauce – 2 tablespoons
- Cornflour – 1 tablespoon
- Mirin – 1 tablespoon
- Crushed garlic cloves – 2
- Sesame oil – 1 teaspoon
- Dried chili flakes – 1 teaspoon

Directions

1. Heat the frying oil in a large wok. Put almonds and fry for a minute until you see a brown color. After browning, scoop them using a slotted spoon onto a plate.

2. Next, generously season the chicken before putting it in the wok. Fry it for 3-4 minutes until it browns. After the fourth minute, scoop and transfer to a plate.

3. Don't wipe the wok and proceed to put broccoli, carrot and baby corn and cook for the next 4-5 minutes until they all look scorched. Stir in red pepper and ginger and let it fry for 2 minutes.

4. As the food fries, take a small bowl and combine cornflour with 100ml cold water. Mix until it's even. Add mirin, soy, garlic, sesame oil and chili flakes into the corn flour mixture and mix them once more.

5. Back to the wok, put the chicken and almonds followed by the sauce you prepared in steps 6 and 7, spring onions, and baby pak choy.

6. Let it to simmer gently for another 3-4 minutes until the onions and pak choy become tender. Make sure the chicken cooks through as the sauce thickens by stirring. When it is all ready, turn off the heat and serve.

14. Cashew Chicken Ding with Celery, Jicama (Mexican Turnip) and Red Bell Pepper

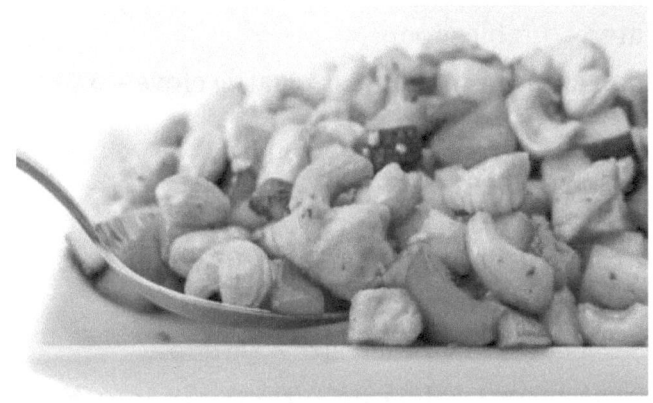

Cook this one if you have a lovely weekend out with nothing much to do. It will take you some hours before meal time.

Cooking time: 2hours
Serving: 2 to 4

Ingredients

- Chicken breast, ¾-inch dices – ¾ pounds
- Soy sauce – 1 teaspoon
- Vegetable or canola oil – 8 teaspoons, divided
- White pepper powder – ¼ teaspoon
- Shaoxing wine – 1 teaspoon
- Kosher salt – ¼ teaspoon, add more if not enough
- Sugar – ¼ teaspoon
- Cornstarch – ¾ teaspoon

Sauce ingredients

- Soy sauce – 1 teaspoon
- Cornstarch – ½ teaspoon
- Toasted sesame oil – 1 teaspoon
- Water – 1 tablespoon
- Finely minced medium size garlic clove – 1

Stir-fry ingredients

- Button mushrooms or stemmed cremini. Cut into ¾-inch dices – 6 ounces
- Celery, cut into ¾-inch size – ½ cup
- Peeled Jicama (Mexican turnip), cut into ¾-inch dices – 1 cup
- Zucchini (courgette), ¾-inch diced – 1 cup
- Toasted cashew nuts – 1 cup, divided
- Stemmed and seeded red bell pepper, cut into ¾-inch sizes – 1, fit ½ cup
- Cooked white rice, ready to serve

Directions

1. Take a medium bowl and thoroughly mix the following: chicken cubes, two teaspoons of oil, Shaoxing wine, soy sauce, sugar, white pepper, cornstarch and salt. Refrigerate the mixture for at least 30 minutes. If you are looking forward to preparing the next day, have it stay refrigerated overnight.

2. To prepare the sauce, combine the ingredients listed for the sauce part and mix thoroughly. Remove the refrigerated chicken mixture 5 minutes before cooking.

3. In the meantime, get a wok and heat two teaspoons of oil until it's smoking hot. Put the chicken in the wok and make sure the pieces lie on the wok surface with the help of a spatula. Cook without moving the meat for a minute. The chicken should turn brown at the bottom.

4. Now, start to stir until the chicken gets cooked through. That should take you 3-4 minutes. At this point, the meat is ready. Put it in a bowl or plate and set it aside.

5. Without wiping the wok, heat another two teaspoons of oil over high heat until it smokes. Add mushrooms and stir-fry for two minutes. They should release some liquid before seasoning with salt. After seasoning, continue stir-frying until the whole liquid evaporates which should take another 2 minutes or so.

6. When the liquid is gone, put the mushrooms in a bowl and place them aside. With the wok in the same condition, put two more teaspoons of oil and heat high until it smokes. At smoking point, add celery, jicama, and zucchini.

7. Cook and stir for about 3 minutes until the jicama slightly browns. After the jicama browns, add the red bell pepper and salt. Cook for two more minutes until the bell pepper slightly tenders.

8. Now, it's time to put the mushrooms back as you cook and stir for another minute. Return the chicken to the wok and stir properly. When the chicken mixes with wok contents, stir the sauce too using a small spoon and pour it into the wok.

9. Stir and cook the meat together with the sauce for a minute or until the sauce thickens. When thickened, turn off the heat and add toasted cashews (¾ cup) as you stir. Put the wok contents on a serving plate. Drizzle the remaining cashews and serve immediately with rice.

15. General Tso Chicken

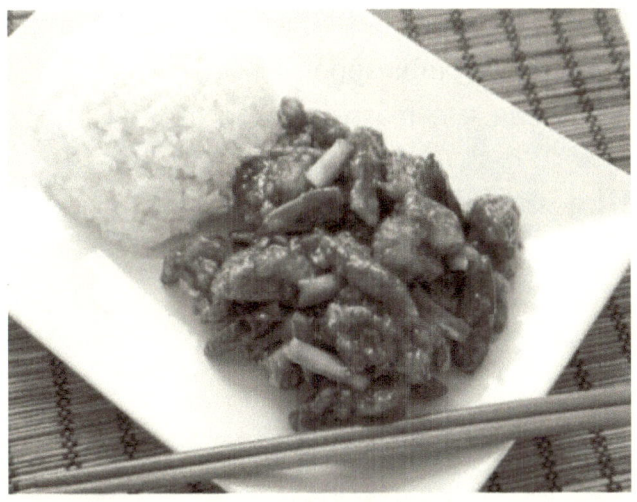

You may probably have seen this in your favorite joint displaying all-sweet. You can still make it in your home and still match what the restaurant has to offer.

Cooking time: varies
Serving: 4 to 6

Ingredients

- Vegetable or canola oil – 1 ½ quarts (about 48 ounces)
- White rice, steamed to serve

Marinade ingredients

- Skinless and boneless chicken thighs, cut into ½-inch pieces – 1 pound
- Dark soy sauce – 2 tablespoons

- Egg white – 1
- Vodka, 80-proof – 2 tablespoons
- Shaoxing wine (Chinese rice wine) – 2 tablespoons
- Cornstarch – 3 tablespoons
- Baking soda – ¼ teaspoon

Dry coating ingredients

- Cornstarch – ½ cup
- Flour – ½ cup
- Kosher salt – ½ teaspoon

Sauce ingredients

- Shaoxing wine – 2 tablespoons
- Dark soy sauce – 3 tablespoons
- Distilled white vinegar or Chinese rice vinegar – 2 tablespoons
- Sugar – 4 tablespoons
- Bought or homemade low-sodium chicken stock – 3 tablespoons
- Cornstarch – 1 tablespoon
- Sesame seed oil, roasted – 1 teaspoon
- Vegetable or canola oil – 2 teaspoons
- Fresh and minced ginger, 1-inch piece – 2 teaspoons
- Two medium garlic cloves, minced – 2 teaspoons
- Scallions, one bottom part minced – 2 teaspoons; White pieces only, cut into 1-inch lengths – 6 to 8
- Small and dried chili pepper – 8

Directions

Preparing the marinade

1. Take a large bowl and beat the egg white until it foams lightly. Add wine, soy sauce, and vodka to the bowl and whisk to mix.

2. Pour half of the mixture into a separate bowl and set it aside. To the remaining marinade, add cornstarch and baking soda and whisk.

3. Put chicken in the bowl with cornstarch and make sure they are well coated. You can use fingers to do so. Cover the composition with a plastic wrap and place somewhere, aside.

Preparing the dry coat

1. In another bowl, mix the following: cornstarch, flour, ½ teaspoon of salt and baking powder. Whisk until you get a smooth mixture.

2. Take the marinade you poured into a separate bowl and mix with what you prepared in step 1 until you have a coarse and clumpy result before setting aside.

Preparing the sauce

1. Mix the following in a small bowl: wine, soy sauce, vinegar, sugar, chicken stock cornstarch and sesame seed oil.

2. Use a fork to stir until all cornstarch gets dissolved with no lumps. After mixing, set it aside.

Meal preparation

1. Take a wok or large skillet and put oil, ginger, garlic, red chilies and the minced scallions. Use medium heat at this point. Cook as you stir for about 3 minutes until fragrance. Make sure they don't turn brown.

2. Stir the sauce mixture before adding it to the wok. Make sure everything gets out of the bowl by scrapping the contents sunk at the bottom. Cook and stir for a minute or until the sauce boils and thickens. At this point, add the scallion pieces.

3. Stir a bit for the scallions to mix then stop cooking and transfer the made sauce to a bowl. Don't wipe the wok or skillet. Heat the peanut and oil in the wok. As the oil heats, it's time for the next steps. Taking one piece at a time, remove the chicken from marinade and toss it in the dry coat.

4. To make sure every piece is thoroughly coated, toss the chicken in the dry coat using your hands and make sure you press the mixture onto the chicken for adherence.

5. Still, one piece at a time, take the chicken from the dry coat, shaking the excess, and carefully put them in the wok/skillet. Don't drop meat pieces.

6. After adding all the chicken, cook and use long chopsticks (or whatever you are comfortable stirring with) to stir after adjusting the temperature to medium (325-375 degrees F).

7. Cook for the next four minutes until the chicken is cooked through and looks crispy. Switch off the heat briefly and transfer the meat to a bowl lined with paper towel for draining purposes.

8. When drained, turn the heat on and return the chicken to the empty wok together with the sauce. Start tossing and use a rubber spatula to fold until the pieces have a thorough coating. Turn off the heat after coating and serve immediately with rice.

16. Sichuan Kung Pao Chicken

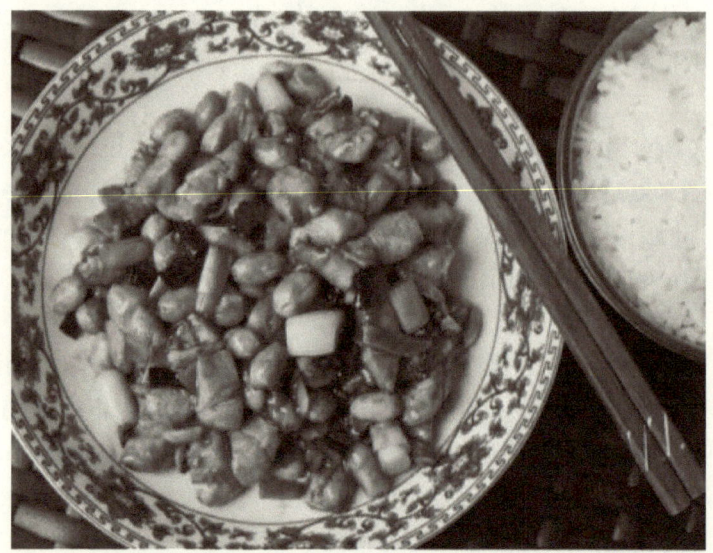

For the Kung Pao recipe, the difference between the one you may be aware of and this one is mild so, it's a weeknight dish worth trying.

Cooking time: 15 minutes
Serving: 2

Ingredients

Chicken ingredients

- Small and boneless chicken breasts, ½-inch cubed – 2, 6 ounces each (170 grams)
- Light soy sauce – 2 teaspoons
- Shaoxing wine – 1 teaspoon
- Kosher salt – 1 pinch, preferably large

- Cornstarch – 2 teaspoons

Sauce ingredients

- Chinkiang vinegar (Chinese black rice vinegar) – 2 tablespoons
- Honey – 1 tablespoon
- Light soy sauce – 2 teaspoons
- Shaoxing wine – 1 tablespoon
- Cornstarch – ½ teaspoon
- Low-sodium chicken stock or water (choose between the two)

Stir-fry ingredients

- Stemmed and seeded small red chili peppers, cut using scissors into ½-inch pieces – 6-12
- Vegetable oil – 3 tablespoons
- Stemmed and seeded Sichuan peppercorns – 1 teaspoon
- Peeled and grated ginger or cut into small matchsticks – 1-inch knob
- Medium size garlic cloves, thinly sliced – 4
- Roasted peanuts – ¾ cup (150 grams or 5 ounces)
- Scallions, pale green and white parts, cut into ½-inch pieces – 6

Directions

Chicken preparation

1. In a small bowl, mix chicken with soy sauce, wine, salt, and cornstarch.

2. After an even mixture, add the meat pieces and turn them well until you get an even coat with a thin film of the resulting paste. After a proper coating, set them aside.

Sauce preparation

1. In another small bowl mix the following: cornstarch, vinegar, honey, soy sauce and wine.

2. Use a fork to stir until there are no cornstarch clumps.

Stir-fry preparation

1. Take a large wok/skillet and pour a little oil and don't heat. Instead, rub it in the wok or skillet using a paper towel.

2. Now, it's time to heat until the wok smokes then add the remaining oil which should be followed by the Sichuan peppercorns and chili. Stir-fry to get the fragrance which should take you about 5 minutes. Make sure they do not get burnt.

3. After smelling the aroma, put the chicken immediately and stir-fry until the pink spots disappear. It should take you 45 sec-1 ½ minutes.

4. When the pink disappears, add ginger and garlic and stir-fry for another 10 seconds or until fragrant. Follow by putting the peanuts and scallions and stir for 30 seconds.

5. After stirring the scallions, add the sauce ingredients. Continue stir-frying for a minute or so, until all they get an even coat as the chicken cooks through. If necessary, add a tablespoon of water so that the sauce does not clump. Is it ready? Serve immediately with the prepared rice.

17. Chicken with Oyster Sauce and Mushrooms

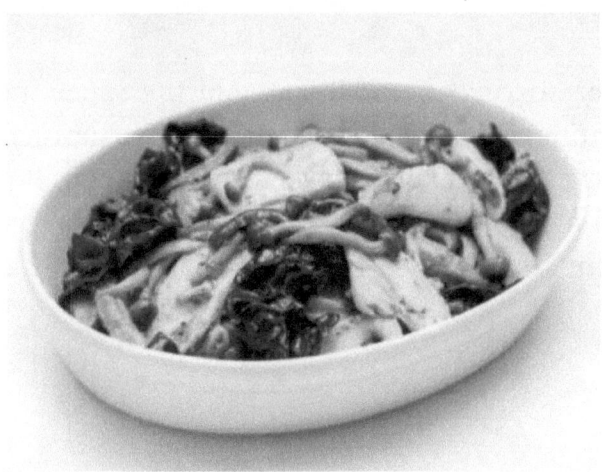

With water-velveted chicken, this easy recipe is a tender and silky meat guarantee. Adding dried and fresh mushrooms define the flavor and texture.

Cooking time: 50 minutes
Serving: 2

Ingredients

Velveted chicken ingredients

- Chicken breast, 1/8-inch slices
- Cornstarch – 2 teaspoons
- Egg white – 1 tablespoon
- Kosher salt – ¼ teaspoon
- Rice wine (Chinese) – 2 teaspoons
- Vegetable or canola oil – 1 teaspoon

- Water – 6 cups

Stir-fry and sauce ingredients

- A variety of mixed mushrooms (what you prefer), ¼-inch thick slices – ½ pound
- Sesame oil – 1 teaspoon
- Cornstarch – 1 teaspoon
- Soy sauce – 1 teaspoon
- Oyster sauce – 2 teaspoons
- Vegetable or canola oil – 2 tablespoons, divided
- Medium and finely minced garlic clove – 1
- Wood ear mushrooms (also known as jelly ear), rehydrated for 15 minutes in warm water then drained, half the large pieces – ¼ cup
- Water – 2 tablespoons
- Cooked white rice. Ready to serve

Directions

Preparing velveted chicken

1. Get a small bowl and thoroughly mix the following: cornstarch, egg white, salt and rice wine.

2. Take another bowl and put the chicken meat. Add the mixture made in step 1 and combine by tossing then place the meat in a refrigerator for 30 minutes.

3. After the ½ hour wait, take a wok and heat the water to boil. At boiling point, add oil.

4. Put the refrigerated chicken and cook as you separate the pieces using a spatula or chopsticks for 40 seconds. The chicken should have an outer white color but still raw inside.

5. Drain the chicken using a bowl-shaped strainer to shake it off before setting aside. After emptying the wok, clean it by wiping.

Stir-fry and sauce preparation

1. Take a small bowl and mix the following: sesame oil, cornstarch, soy sauce, garlic, oyster sauce, and water. When the mixture is ready, get a wok and strongly heat a tablespoon of vegetable. When hot, add the mixed mushrooms and season them using salt. Cook by tossing and stirring for about three minutes until the mushrooms release water.

2. After the water release, add the wood ear mushrooms (jelly ear mushrooms). Cook then for about 5 minutes until the mushrooms attain a brown color. Are they browned? Transfer the mushrooms to a plate and wipe the wok.

3. In a clean wok, put the remaining vegetable oil (1 tablespoon) into the wok and heat strongly to smoke. Add chicken and stir-fry for two minutes until it is almost cooked through. When the meat appears ready, put the mushrooms back in the wok and stir so that they mix with the chicken meat.

4. Now, it's time to add the sauce. Stir it before adding to the wok. Toss together with the meat and mushrooms for a minute or so until you get a thick mixture. When ready, put the cooked stew on a serving plate and serve with the prepared white rice.

18. Honey Nut Chicken

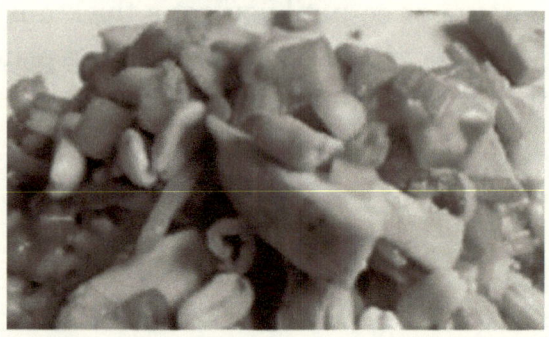

Here is an elegant dish with celery and orange honey sauce for a midweek lunch or dinner.

Cooking time: 20 minutes
Serving: 4

Ingredients

- Boneless chicken breast, cut into strips – 1 ½ pounds
- Chopped celery stalks – 2
- Peanut oil – 2 teaspoons
- Peeled carrots, sliced diagonally – 2
- Orange juice – ¾ cup
- Cornstarch – 1 tablespoon
- Honey – 1 tablespoon
- Light soy sauce – 3 tablespoons
- Cashew peanuts – ¼ cup
- Fresh and minced ginger root – 1 teaspoon
- Minced green onions – ¼ cup

Directions

1. Take a small bowl and thoroughly mix orange juice with cornstarch. Add honey, soy sauce, and ginger. After an even mixture, set it aside.

2. It's time for the wok. Heat a teaspoon of oil over high heat. At smoking point, add celery and carrots and cook as you stir for 3 minutes.

3. Still in the wok, add one more teaspoon of oil followed by an immediate addition of chicken and stir-fry for another 5 minutes.

4. Stir the sauce mixture made in step 1 and add it to the wok. Switch the heat to medium and cook to get a thick result.

5. Top the stew with green onions and cashew peanuts and switch off the heat before serving.

19. Garden Chicken

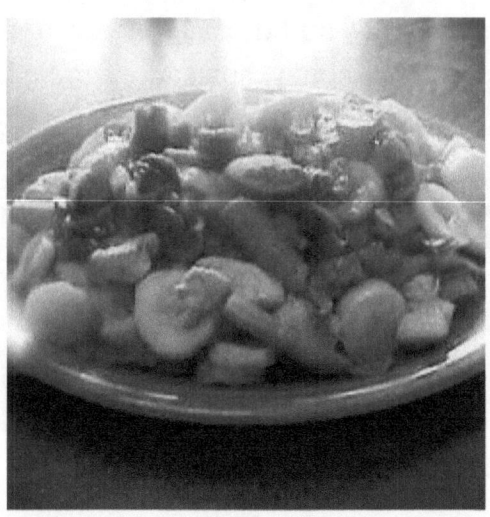

Another one to serve with rice or salad greens is the garden chicken, but it is somewhat a mean recipe since you can only enjoy it alone. With whole pecans and garden vegetables quickly fried with little oil, you have a mouthwatering method that you can only share by telling the idea.

Cooking time: 35 minutes
Serving: 1

Ingredients

- Boneless chicken breasts, cut into strips – 4 halves
- Extra virgin olive oil (made from raw olive juice) – 1 tablespoon
- Small chopped onion – 1
- Carrots, cut into long strips – 1 cup
- Fresh and sliced mushrooms – 1 cup

- Yellow summer squash (harvested immature), peeled and cut into 1-inch pieces – 2
- Peeled Zucchini squash, 1-inch rounds – 1
- Black pepper, ground and coarse – 1 teaspoon
- Halved pecans – ½ cup

Directions

1. Take a wok/nonstick skillet and coat the bottom part lightly with oil. Using medium heat, heat the wok or skillet and put the chicken strips. Cook and stir the meat until you see a light brown color.

2. After browning, add onions and carrots and continue cooking for 3 minutes. Now, it's time to add zucchini, mushrooms, and squash and keep cooking as you stir until the squash starts to soften.

3. When the squash seems to soften, add the pecans and season the wok contents with a teaspoon of pepper. Toss for 2-3 minutes and then switch off the heat once the food is ready. Serve the chicken with salad greens or rice.

20. Avocado Chicken

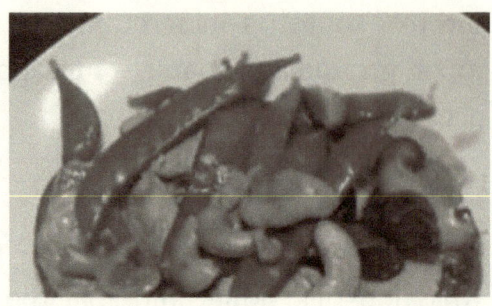

When combined with snow peas and chicken, the avocado has an exceptional taste. One thing you need to note though, unripe avocados will serve you best since they don't mush as you cook. Try serving with rice and comment later.

Cooking time: 40 minutes
Serving: 4

Ingredients

- Boneless chicken breasts, cut into bite-size pieces – 4 halves
- Firm but ripe avocados, peeled, seed removed, and cut into large chunks - 2
- Soy sauce – ¼ cup
- Chicken broth – ½ cup
- Minced garlic clove – 1
- Cornstarch – 1 tablespoon
- Vegetable oil – 1 tablespoon
- Cremini mushrooms, stemmed and thinly sliced – 2 cups
- Snow peas (Chinese peas) – 2 cups

- Green onions, cut into 1-inch pieces – 4 bunches

Directions

1. Start by taking a bowl and mix the following: chicken broth, cornstarch, soy sauce, and garlic. Stir until the cornstarch becomes smooth before setting aside. Put oil in a wok or a large skillet and heat using medium-to-high temperature until the oil shimmers.

2. When the oil is shimmering hot, put the chicken pieces in the wok. Start to cook as you stir for about 5 minutes until the pink color disappears.

3. When the meat is no longer pink, remove it from the wok and set it aside in a bowl. While the wok is still hot, put the snow peas and cook for three minutes until they become light green and crisp.

4. Add oil, green onions, and mushrooms. Start tossing for about 5 minutes until the mushrooms become tender, and the juice is almost evaporated but not gone. If there is excess juice after the 5 minutes, pour it off. Once all the liquid is out, add the chicken to the vegetables and switch the heat to medium before stirring briefly.

5. It's time to add the sauce. If it's thick, stir it before adding to the wok. After the sauce, stir in the avocado gently and let it bubble for 3 minutes, or until the sauce thickens. Stir again to make sure the sauce coats everything before turning of the heat and serving.

21. Orange Chicken

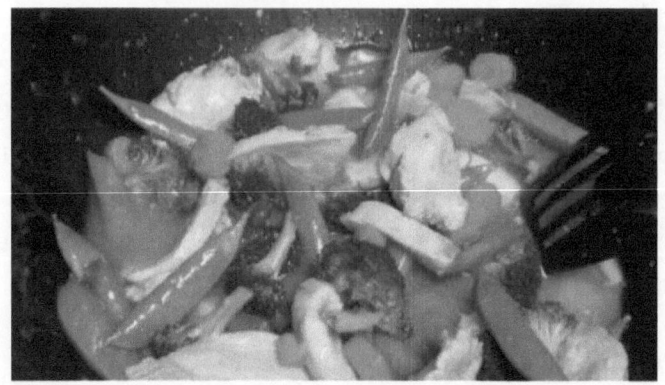

Cooking time: 40 minutes
Serving: 4

Ingredients

- Boneless chicken breasts, thinly sliced – 4 halves
- Orange juice – ½ cup
- Chopped garlic cloves – 3
- Soy sauce – 3 tablespoons
- Ginger, ground – 1 teaspoon
- Grated orange zest (grated orange skin without peeling) – 1 tablespoon
- Vegetable oil – 3 tablespoons
- Crushed red pepper – ½ teaspoon (optional)
- Chicken broth – ½ cup
- Frozen stir-fry vegetables – 16 ounces (1 package)
- Cornstarch – 2 tablespoons
- Sugar snap peas – 1 cup
- Sliced carrot – 1 cup

- Broccoli florets – 1 cup

Directions

1. In a bowl, mix the following thoroughly: soy sauce, orange juice, orange zest, garlic, red pepper flakes, and ginger. After mixing, take a wok or a large skillet and heat oil over medium to high temperature.

2. When hot, put the mixture you prepared in the wok, slowly followed by the meat. Cook and stir for 7-10 minutes until the pink color disappears from the chicken meat and the juices become clear.

3. After the 10th minute, switch the heat to low and take another bowl which you will use to whisk cornstarch and chicken broth together.

4. After making an even mixture, put it in the wok in small amounts and stir after every input until the sauce thickens as preferred.

5. When the sauce thickens, put the frozen vegetables, broccoli, snap peas and carrot in the wok and stir to mix. Continue cooking and stirring until the veggies are somehow soft which should take you another 7-10 minutes. When everything is ready, switch off the heat and serve with hot rice.

22. Duck with Ginger and Greens

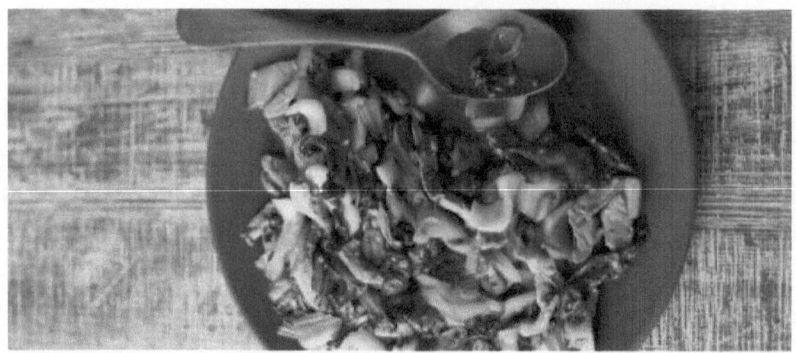

If you love duck meat, then this stir-fry recipe will be easy to make not to mention how well it rhymes with ginger and greens.

Cooking time: 15 minutes
Serving: 4

Ingredients

- Skinless duck breasts, cut into thin strips – 2 halves
- Groundnut oil
- Sliced red chili – 1
- Finely chopped ginger – 1 tablespoon
- Sliced Pak choi – 500 grams
- Honey – 1 tablespoon
- Chopped spring onions – 1 cup
- Soy sauce – 1 teaspoon
- Corn flour – 1 teaspoon
- Oyster sauce – 2 tablespoons

Directions

1. Heat the wok strongly and proceed to add two teaspoons of oil. After the oil, slowly dip the duck breasts and stir for 2 minutes. Are two minutes over? Scoop them out to a bowl and set aside.

2. Once the meat is out, add a teaspoon of oil to the wok. Put chili, ginger, pak choi and most of the spring onions. Cook until the choi loses turgidity. After noting pak choi's water release, sprinkle or drizzle the following in the wok: honey, soy and oyster sauces.

3. Once the honey and sauces are in, put the meat back in the wok and let it bubble for a minute. You won't be stirring since you have something to do in the next step.

4. As the meat cooks, quickly take another bowl and mix corn flour with two teaspoons of cold water until you get a smooth texture.

5. Add the mixture prepared above to the meat. Now, begin to stir until the sauce becomes glossy. When the meat and sauce are ready, switch off the heat. Before you serve, sprinkle the remaining spring onions.

Chapter 3

Stir-Fry Beef Recipes

Beef is a typical dish to many but preparing it in the wok needs the right expertise. For most of the recipes that you'll come across in this chapter, you need meat from animals' sides with no bones. Remember to cut it into bite sizes before tenderizing and stirring.

Most of the recipes that I have included take less time amounting to minutes, small pieces will cook through within the stipulated time. If you are still wondering where to get the specified meat, you can go for beef from any part as long as it's boneless and ease your worries in the long run.

23. Crispy Chili Beef

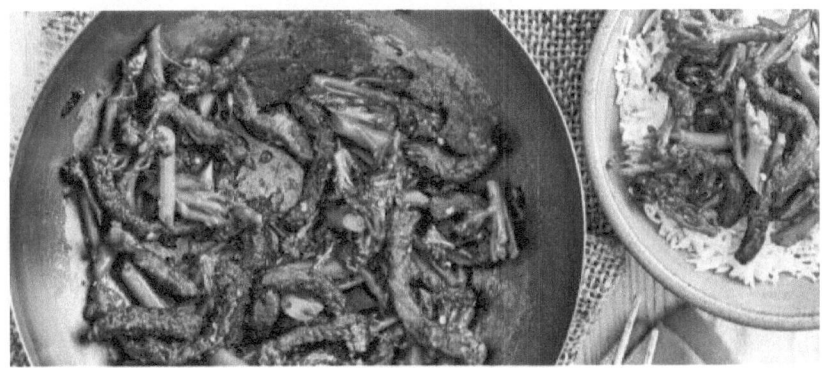

Cooking time: 20-30 minutes
Serving: 2

Ingredients

- Broccolini (tenderstem), cut into small pieces – 150 grams
- Chinese five-spice (a mixture of 5 Chinese-origin spices) – 2 teaspoons
- Corn flour – 2 tablespoons
- Sunflower/groundnut oil
- Sirloin (meat from animal's back), trim off the fat and cut into thin strips – 2 steaks
- Crushed garlic clove – 1
- Grated ginger – 1 chunk
- Dried chili flakes – ½ teaspoon
- Brown sugar – 2 teaspoons
- Soy sauce and brown sugar mixture – combine 2 teaspoons each
- Rice vinegar – 2 teaspoons

Directions

1. Boil some water in a pot and put broccolini when it begins to boil. Let it cook for a minute before draining the water and setting the cut pieces aside.

2. After preparing broccolini, take a small bowl and mix five-spice with corn flour. Once you get an even mixture, toss the steak into the bowl's combination and make sure you achieve a proper coating before taking the wok.

3. In a wok or a heavy non-stick frying pan, heat a small pool of oil over medium to high heat. When the oil is hot, add the steak and fry until it attains a dark golden color.

4. When you finally note the meat's color change, remove it and transfer to a bowl as you drain some of the oil after each scoop. The remaining oil in the wok/pan should be about a teaspoon.

5. Add garlic, chili flakes, and ginger to the oil you saved in the wok. Cook for a minute before putting broccolini. Toss for another minute until the tenderstem is heated through.

6. After the tossing minute, put the steak back and add the rice vinegar and soy sauce. Make sure everything coats before turning off the heat. Serve the beef with rice.

24. Beef and Black Bean

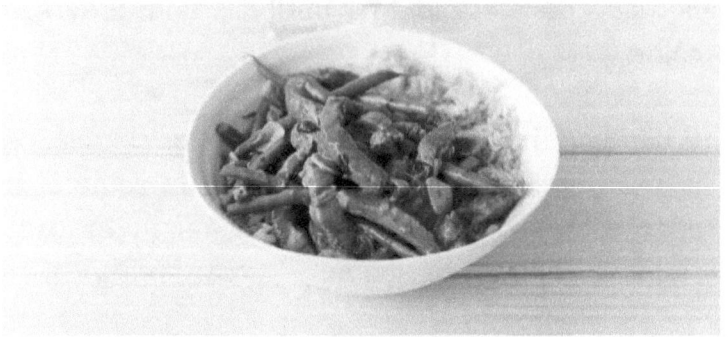

With less than 300 calories and plenty of flavors, this recipe results to healthier food intake as you look forward to ignoring the regular takeaway.

Cooking time: 10 minutes
Serving: 2

Ingredients

- Cube or minute steak, cut into strips – 300 grams
- Grated ginger – 2cm piece
- Finely sliced garlic cloves – 2
- Trimmed and briefly cooked green beans – 2 handfuls
- Black bean sauce (or one with chili) – 4 tablespoons
- Cooking oil
- Cooked brown rice to serve

Directions

1. Take a wok and put a tablespoon of oil. Heat the oil strongly before adding ginger and garlic. Follow by

putting beef in the wok and cook until the meat starts to brown.

2. At browning point, add the green beans and stir-fry for a minute. As you stir, add the bean sauce and splash some water. After the water splash, move everything by stirring to get an even coat.

3. Keep stirring as you let the meat cook for 1-2 minutes before removing the wok from heat. At this point, it's now ready to serve with the cooked rice.

25. Beef with Chinese Broccoli

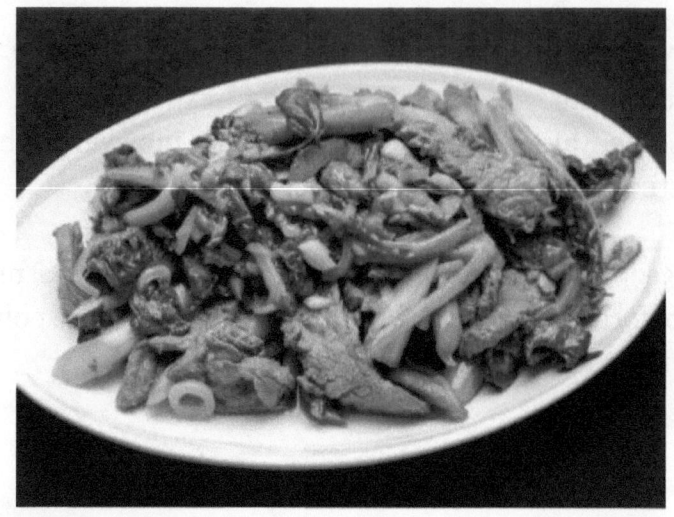

Cooking time: 1 hour
Serving: 2-4

Ingredients

Beef and marinade ingredients

- Beefsteak (from animal's sides), cut into 1/8-inch thick slices – ¾ pounds
- Shaoxing wine – ½ teaspoon
- Soy sauce – ½ teaspoon
- Vegetable/canola oil – 2 teaspoons
- Kosher salt – ½ teaspoon
- Cornstarch – ½ teaspoon
- Sugar – ¼ teaspoon
- Ground white pepper – ¼ teaspoon

Sauce ingredients

- Sesame oil – 1 teaspoon
- Soy sauce – 1 teaspoon
- Oyster sauce – 2 teaspoons
- Cornstarch – 1 teaspoon
- Water – 2 tablespoons

Stir-fry ingredients

- Chinese broccoli, cut into 2-3 pieces diagonally – ½ pound
- Sliced shallots – 2
- Vegetable/canola oil – 2 tablespoons
- Chopped garlic cloves into relatively large pieces – 8

Directions

1. Take a medium bowl and combine all ingredients in the beef marinade section. Mix them thoroughly before setting the bowl aside to let the mixture stand for 30 minutes at room temperature.

2. As you wait, take another bowl and combine the ingredients in the sauce section. Mix them well before setting aside. When the 30-minute period is over, take a wok and fill it halfway with water. Season the water with salt and leave it to boil.

3. At boiling point, add Chinese broccoli and cook for a minute or until you reach a crisp-tender state. After the minute or so, drain the broccoli and set it aside in a

bowl or plate. Wipe the wok and then add a tablespoon of oil. Place it over high heat and let it smoke.

4. At smoking point, add beef and spread it out to an even layer in the wok and using chopsticks or a spatula. Cook without moving the beef for a minute. The beef should be light brown at the bottom before going to the next step. Start stirring and don't stop as you cook for two more minutes until the beef cooks halfway. At this point, transfer the beef to a bowl and set aside.

5. In the empty wok, add a tablespoon of oil and heat vigorously to smoke. At smoking point, put garlic and shallots. Start cooking as you stir continuously for a minute until they soften.

6. Now, it's time to add Chinese broccoli. After the addition, frequently stir for a minute before you season with salt. After seasoning, put the beef back in the wok and toss to get a nice combination.

7. After tossing, get the sauce. Stir it before putting in the wok. Make sure you aim it at the center as you pour.

8. Mix the meat and sauce for coating purposes. Keep cooking as you stir for a minute until the sauce starts to thicken. Upon thickening, immediately transfer the cooked meat to a platter and serve with cooked white rice.

26. Beef with Snap Peas and Oyster Sauce

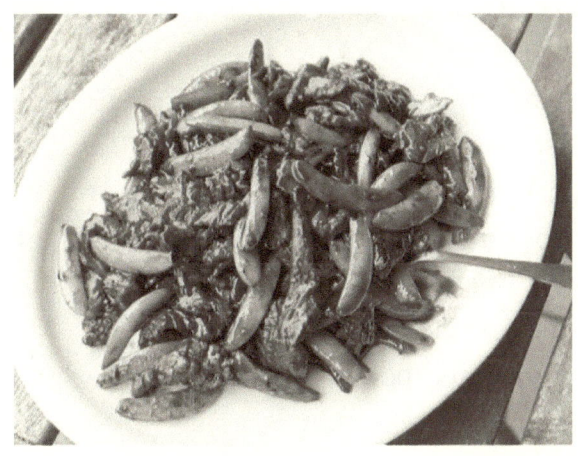

In this quick stir-fry recipe, you need a steak of beef meat that is flappy (flattened and 'wavy') as the primary dish with snap peas adding more to the taste and appearance.

Cooking time: 30 minutes
Serving: 4

Ingredients

Beef ingredients

- Thinly sliced steak of flap meat – 1 pound
- Sugar – ½ teaspoon
- Kosher salt – ½ teaspoon
- Shaoxing wine – 1 teaspoon
- Dark soy sauce – 1 teaspoon
- Baking soda – 1/8 teaspoon

- Toasted sesame oil (roasted) – ½ teaspoon
- Cornstarch – ½ teaspoon

Stir-fry ingredients

- Shaoxing wine – 2 tablespoon
- Dark soy sauce – 2 tablespoons
- Oyster sauce – ¼ cup
- Low-sodium chicken stock (homemade or from the store) – ¼ cup
- Toasted sesame oil – 1 teaspoon
- Sugar – 2 tablespoons
- Cornstarch – 1 teaspoon
- Trimmed snap peas – 1 pound
- Finely minced medium garlic cloves – 2
- Vegetable or canola oil – 3 tablespoons
- Finely minced fresh ginger – 2 teaspoons
- Finely minced scallion, white and light green parts – 1

Directions

1. In a small bowl, combine everything in the beef ingredients section. Toss the combination to mix and leave it for the next 20 minutes.

2. Meanwhile, in another bowl, stir to combine everything in the stir-fry ingredients section. Set it aside too after a thorough mixing chore.

3. After the mixing task, get a wok and heat a tablespoon of oil over high heat until it smokes. After smoking the

oil, put half of the beef in the wok and spread it to achieve a single layer in the wok.

4. Cook without moving the meat for a minute until the sides attached to the wok have a light brown color. After an underneath browning of the meat, start to toss and stir frequently for another minute to cook it lightly through.

5. At this point, put the beef in a bowl and place it aside. Repeat steps and always remember to add a tablespoon of oil for the remaining meat as you repeat.

6. After the light cooking and setting aside beef preparation, wipe the wok and proceed to heat the remaining tablespoon of oil until it's smoking hot.

7. When the oil smokes, put snap peas in the wok. Cook as you stir and toss until they have charred spots but with a bright green coloring.

8. Follow by adding ginger, garlic, and scallions. Continue cooking as you stir until a sweet aroma reaches you. Return the beef to the wok and toss for a good combination.

9. Next, stirring the sauce briefly and add to the wok. Toss and stir continuously for a minute. The sauce should thicken and coat the beef and veggies evenly. Have you coated the meat and vegetables properly? Turn off the heat and serve immediately.

27. Chinese Pepper Steak

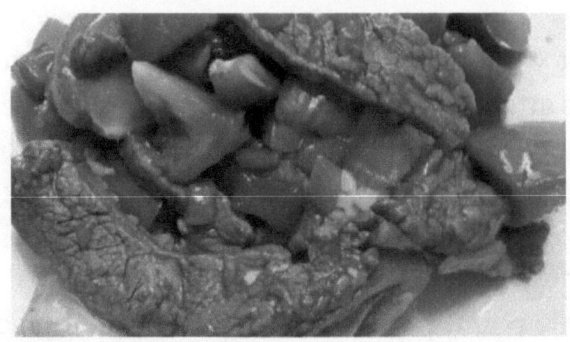

Cooking time: 30 minutes
Serving: 4

Ingredients

- Beef sirloin steak (cut from the abdomen area) – 1 pound
- Soy sauce – ¼ cup
- Cornstarch – 2 tablespoons
- White sugar – 2 tablespoons
- Vegetable oil – 3 tablespoons, divided
- Ground ginger – ½ teaspoon
- Red onion, cut into 1-inch square pieces – 1
- Tomatoes, cut into wedges - 2
- Green bell pepper, cut into 1-inch pieces – 1

Directions

1. First, cut the steak against the grain (against the fiber lining) into ½-inch thick pieces.

2. Next, start preparing the marinade by taking a bowl and thoroughly mixing the following: sugar, soy sauce, ginger, and cornstarch. Make sure all sugar has dissolved, and you have a smooth mixture.

3. Put the beef slices in the marinade and make sure they coat well by stirring. After marinating, it is time to use the wok.

4. In a wok or a large skillet, heat a tablespoon of vegetable oil over medium to high heat. Follow by putting a third of the steak into the oil. Cook by stirring the meat for three minutes, until the beef is all-around brown.

5. In the fourth minute, remove the meat by scooping and set aside. Repeat step 5 for the remaining beef, setting aside each time in the same bowl or plate. Since you are taking a third each time, you will do it twice.

6. While the wok is still hot and unwiped, put all the beef back in. Start stirring and put the onions in the process. Toss the beef and onions for two minutes or so, until the onions start to soften.

7. Now, it's time to add the green pepper and stir. Let it cook as you keep stirring for two minutes. The pepper should turn bright green and start to tender. As the pepper tenderizes, add tomatoes to the mixture. Stir everything and serve when it is ready.

28. Quick Beef Recipe

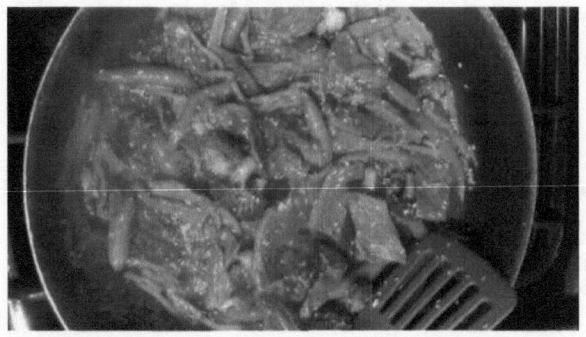

Cooking time: 25 minutes
Serving: 4

Ingredients

- Beef sirloin, cut into 2-inch strips – 1 pound
- Broccoli florets – ½ cup
- Vegetable oil – 2 tablespoons
- Red bell pepper, cut matchstick-wise – 1
- Chopped green onion – 1
- Thinly sliced carrots – 2
- Minced garlic – 1 teaspoon
- Toasted sesame seeds – 2 tablespoons
- Soy sauce – 2 tablespoons

Directions

1. In a large wok/skillet, heat the vegetable oil using the medium to high heat. With the oil hot, stir in the beef and cook for 3-4 minutes until it attains a brown color.

2. After the browning gesture, scoop the meat out and put it in a bowl. In an empty wok, add broccoli, carrots, bell pepper, garlic and green onions to the wok and aim at the center as you put them. Cook as you stir the veggies for two minutes.

3. When they start to become tender, return the beef and stir together with the vegetables to mix everything. Is the mixture okay? Season the meat using sesame seeds and soy sauce.

4. Now, cook and stir for another 2 minutes until the vegetables seem to tenderize. When the veggies are ready and the beef is cooked through, turn off the heat and serve.

29. Orange Zest Beef (Spicy)

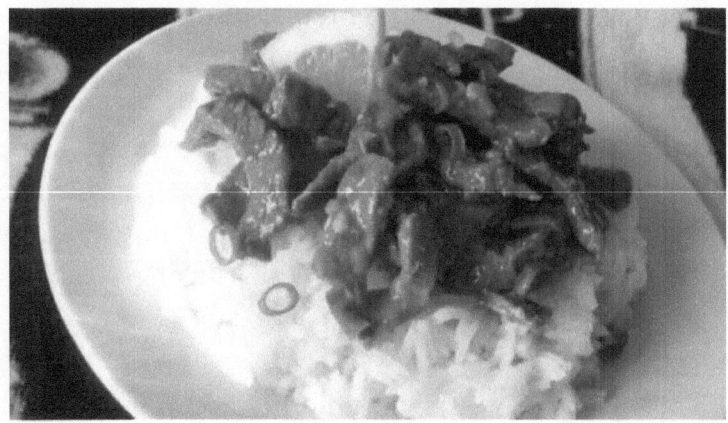

It takes more than an hour to prepare this recipe so, it's a good idea to consider it during the weekend. If you don't like too much fat, it's low in this recipe.

Cooking time: 2 hours
Serving: 4

Ingredients

- Beef tenderloin, ½-inch strips – 1 pound
- Seasoned rice vinegar (sugar and salt added) – ¼ cup
- Orange juice – ¼ cup
- Hot chili paste – 1 tablespoon
- Soy sauce – 2 tablespoons
- Brown sugar – 1 tablespoon
- Garlic cloves, minced – 2
- Cornstarch – 1 teaspoon
- Grated orange zest (orange peeling) – 2 tablespoons
- Cooking spray

- Sliced green onions, separate white and top parts – 1 bunch
- Fresh and ground black pepper – 1 pinch or as preferred
- Salt to taste

Directions

1. In a large bowl, thoroughly mix the following: beef, rice vinegar, orange juice, soy sauce, brown sugar, garlic and hot chili paste. After mixing, cover the bowl and refrigerate for an hour.

2. After an hour's wait, strain the beef using a colander over a clean bowl and let the meat to thoroughly drain for five minutes. Once you're through, put the marinade (mixture prepared in earlier step) aside for the next step.

3. Put cornstarch and water in the marinade. Dissolve the cornstarch by whisking, then set aside when it's ready.

4. Now, it's time to start cooking. Spray a skillet or a non-stick frying pan with cooking spray and heat vigorously.

5. When the skillet or pan is hot, put beef and cook without stirring for one minute. When the minute is over, start to mix and keep going for another minute.

6. Still, as you stir after a minute, put orange zest and the white parts from the green onions. Let them cook for 30

seconds and keep stirring. Follow by putting the green parts of the onions together with marinade.

7. Keep stirring as you cook so that the beef is no longer pink inside and also allow the sauce to thicken. It should take you 2-3 minutes. Season with black pepper and salt to taste before you turn off the heat and serve.

30. Sesame Beef

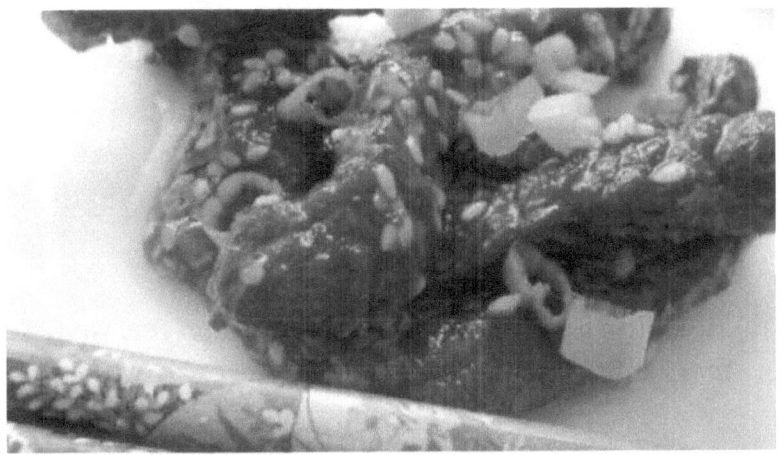

Another one to serve with rice is round steak that is quickly stir-fried with sesame seeds. You can add sesame oil to the marinade if you like the flavor.

Cooking time: 45 minutes
Serving: 4

Ingredients

- Round steak (from animal's rear leg) – 1 pound
- White sugar – 4 tablespoons
- Soy sauce – 4 tablespoons
- Vegetable oil – 4 tablespoons
- Minced garlic cloves – 2
- Sesame seeds – 2 tablespoons
- Chopped green onions – 2

Directions

1. Take a large bowl and mix the following: sugar, garlic, soy sauce, oil, and onions. Once you get an even combination, set the mixture aside.

2. Next, cut the steak into strips and put them in the bowl with the mixture prepared in the first step.

3. Make sure you immerse the meat pieces well. After marinating, cover the bowl and refrigerate for 30 minutes or overnight if you want to prepare the next day.

4. After refrigeration, start to cook the beef in a wok without any oil for five minutes until it turns brown. It should take you 5 minutes.

5. After the fifth minute, add sesame seeds and cook for another 2 minutes. After two minutes are over, remove the wok from heat and serve.

31. Mongolian Beef and Spring Onions

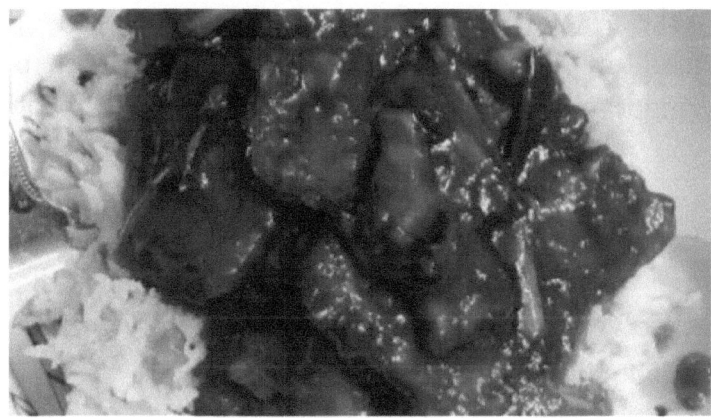

You can serve this soya-based beef with rice noodles or white rice.

Cooking time: 30 minutes
Serving: 4

Ingredients

- Beefsteak (from the sides), sliced to ¼-inch thick pieces against the fiber lining – 1 pound
- Dark brown sugar – 2/3 cup
- Vegetable oil – 2 teaspoons
- Soy sauce – ½ cup
- Finely chopped garlic – 1 tablespoon
- Fresh and grated ginger root – ½ teaspoon
- Water – ½ cup
- Cornstarch – ¼ cup
- Green onions, cut to 2-inch lengths – 2 bunches

Directions

1. Take a saucepan and heat two teaspoons of oil over medium heat. Wait for it to get hot before putting ginger and garlic then stir until fragrant. It should take you 30 seconds.

2. Follow by putting soy sauce, brown sugar, and water to the wok. Switch the heat to high and stir until the sugar dissolves and the sauce boils to slightly thick. It will take you four minutes.

3. Once the sauce seems thick, remove the contents from the wok and set them aside. Switch off the heat before going to the next step.

4. Now that the wok is empty, take a bowl and put beef together with cornstarch. Toss so that the beef can coat with the oil before you let it sit for 10 minutes.

5. After the tenth minute, get ready for the wok. Take it (or a large skillet) and heat vegetable oil to 190 degrees Celsius or until hot.

6. When hot, take the beef, shaking the cornstarch, a few pieces at a time and put it in the hot oil. Briefly stir to cook the meat for two minutes until the edges start to crisp and brown.

7. At this point, the beef is ready for scooping out and putting it onto a plate with paper towels to drain the excess oil. Pour the remaining oil out of the wok/skillet

and then proceed to heat it using medium heat with no oil. Wait for it to get hot and then return the beef and stir briefly.

8. Next, take the reserved sauce, stir it briefly and add to the wok followed by the green onions. Let the mixture boil and cook so that the onions can soften and attain a bright green color. It should take you two minutes before turning off the heat and serving.

32. Black Pepper Beef and Cabbage

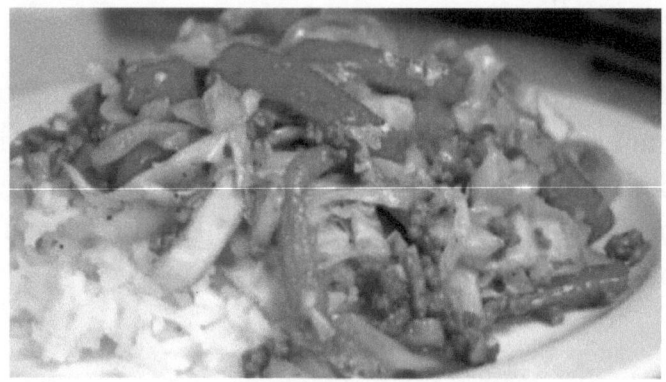

Husbands will love this so make sure there is no one in the list of people to feed when cooking this one. You can serve it with hot steamed rice.

Cooking time: 30 minutes
Serving: 4

Ingredients

- Ground beef – ½ pound
- Vegetable oil – 2 tablespoon
- Small cabbage, shredded – ½ head
- Chopped garlic cloves, chopped – 4
- Soy sauce – 2 tablespoons
- Red bell pepper, cut into strips – 1
- Water (preferably cold) – ½ cup
- Cornstarch – 1 teaspoon
- Ground black pepper – 1 teaspoon
- Salt (optional)

Directions

1. Start by putting oil in a wok/skillet and heating it over medium to high heat. Put garlic in the hot oil and cook briefly for 5 seconds before adding the ground beef.

2. Cook and stir until you get an even brown mixture. After browning, scoop the beef out and drain the excess fat before placing it in a bowl and then returning it to the wok.

3. Start to stir and while in the motion, put cabbage and pepper. Keep cooking until the veggies become tender and the beef becomes fully cooked.

4. Now, it's time to put soy sauce to the wok and stir. Leave the wok a bit and quickly take a bowl to mix water with cornstarch. Mix them well before stirring the mixture in the wok.

5. After adding the cornstarch mixture, season the beef with salt and pepper. Keep stirring for the sauce to thicken. After the sauce thickens, remove the wok from heat and serve.

33. Beef with Tangerine Sauce

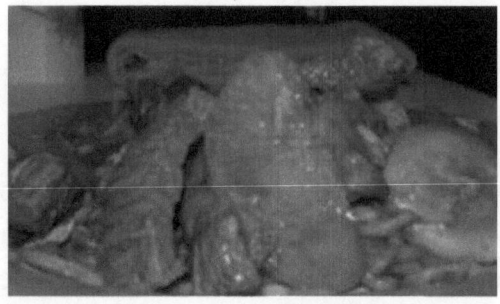

If you do not like the spicy beef, try this one.

Cooking time: 45 minutes
Serving: 4

Ingredients

- Beefsteak (from animal sides), cut diagonally into 2-inch strips – 1 pound
- Dry Chinese noodles – 1 package, 8 ounces
- Sherry (a fortified wine from white grapes) – ¼ cup
- Hoisin sauce – ¼ cup
- Tangerine zest (grate the outer cover while fruit still intact) – 1 teaspoon
- Ground ginger – 1 teaspoon
- Vegetable oil – 4 teaspoons
- Fresh and sliced mushrooms – 1 cup
- Butternut pumpkin, peel, remove the seeds and slice thinly – ½ small head
- Thinly sliced cabbage – 3 cups
- Red onion, large cut into 2-inch strips – 1

- Tangerine, seeded and divided into segments – 1

Directions

1. You should start by preparing the pasta. Fill a pot with water and some salt and bring to boil over high heat. As the water boils, stir the noodles in and let it simmer. Cook as you stir the noodles for 5 minutes so that they can be firm when you bite. When they are ready, rinse and drain before setting them aside.

2. Once the noodles are ready, take a small bowl and whisk the following together: sherry, hoisin sauce, ground pepper and tangerine zest. After whisking, take a wok and heat two teaspoons of vegetable oil over high heat.

3. When the oil is hot, put half of the beef slices and continuously stir for 2-3 minutes until the meat gets a nice brown coat. At this point, remove the beef from the wok using a scoop. Repeat steps for the remaining beef.

4. When the meat is ready, heat the remaining oil (2 teaspoons) and put the onions, mushrooms and butternut squash before stirring them all. Continue stirring for 5-7 minutes until the veggies are crisp but tender and the edges are brown in color.

5. Follow by adding the cabbage. Cook as you stir for another two minutes until they slightly wilt.

6. When the cabbage slightly cooks, switch the heat to medium and stir in the cooked beef, hoisin mixture, and tangerine sections.

7. Once they are all in, cook as you stir for 2-3 minutes until they are all heated through. After the third minute, switch off the heat and immediately serve with the prepared noodles.

Chapter 4

Marine Stir-Fry Recipes

It's time for the wok to do some fishing. In most of the recipes, you can substitute the crustacean, mollusks or fish prescribed with what you like.

34. Shrimp, Eggs and Garlic Chives

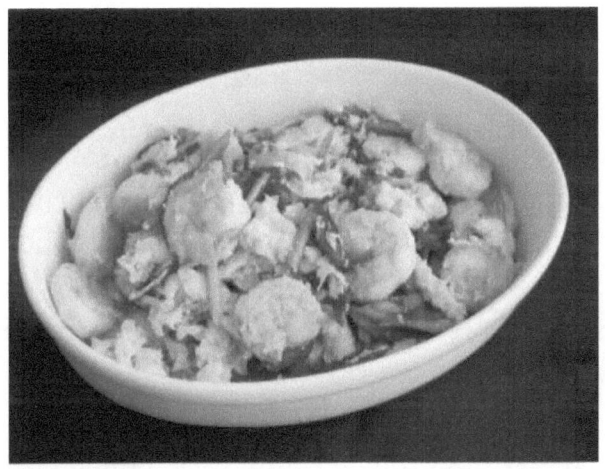

If you cannot access the shrimp, replace it with sliced and roasted pork.

Cooking time: 40 minutes
Serving: 2

Ingredients

- Medium shrimp, keep it shelled and remove the dorsal vein – ½ pound

- Vegetable oil – 2 tablespoons and 1 teaspoon, divided
- Baking soda – 1 teaspoon
- Kosher salt – ½ teaspoon, divide equally
- Large eggs – 4
- Ground white pepper – ½ teaspoon, divide equally
- Milk – 1 tablespoon
- Medium garlic cloves, minced – 2
- Garlic chives (Chinese chives), cut into 1-inch length – almost 1 cup (2 ounces)
- Fresh and minced ginger – 1 teaspoon

Directions

1. Start by taking a medium bowl, put some cold water and immerse the shrimp. After that, pour baking soda and stir. Refrigerate the shrimp in the bowl for 30 minutes. After the ½ hour is over, drain the shrimp and rinse with tap water. Follow by drying it using paper towels.

2. When dry, put the shrimp in a small bowl. Add a teaspoon of oil, salt and one part of the white pepper you divided. Mix them well and set aside before going to the next step. Take another bowl, medium size, and whisk the following together: all the eggs, the remaining salt, and white pepper.

3. Once you get an even mixture, start cooking by heating a tablespoon of oil in a wok until it slightly smokes, over high heat. Once the oil is hot, put the shrimp in and stir for one minute.

4. Proceed to add garlic, garlic chives, and ginger. Stir-fry for another minute for the chives to wilt a little bit. The shrimp should also be lightly cooked after the 60 seconds stirring activity. After the minute is over, transfer the contents to a plate and set aside.

5. Put the remaining oil (1 tablespoon) in the wok and heat until it lightly smokes. Put eggs in the wok and switch the heat to medium. Do not stir the egg so that the bottom layer can form. It should take you 30 seconds.

6. Start to scrape the eggs using a spatula from the sides, moving towards the center of the wok. Keep doing it until the eggs are semisolid and halfway cooked.

7. With the eggs almost cooked, add the shrimp and chives to the wok. Gently stir until the eggs are faintly flowing. At this point, turn off the heat, put the prepared food on a platter and serve immediately.

35. Bang Bang Chili Prawn

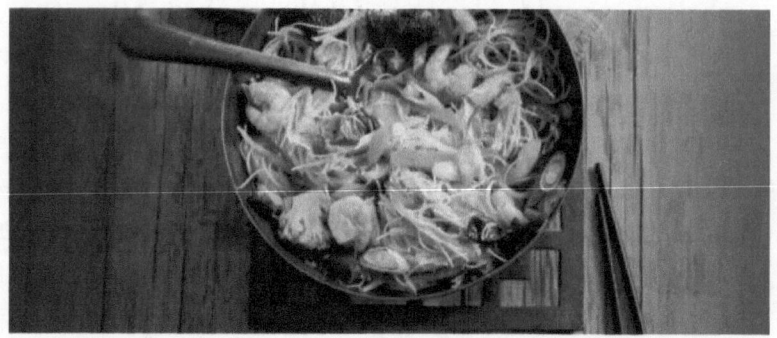

If you want to cook the bang-bang, first attend to the paste preparation a day before cooking the prawn.

Cooking time: 20 minutes
Serving: 4

Ingredients

Bang bang paste ingredients

- Sriracha sauce (or hot sauce) – 1 tablespoon
- Garlic powder – ½ teaspoon
- Brown sugar – 1 teaspoon
- Sweet chili sauce – 5 tablespoons
- Rice vinegar – ½ teaspoon
- Mayo – ½ cup

Other ingredients

- King prawns (or just prawns) – 175 grams (about 0.4 pounds)

- Stir-fry vegetable mix – 285 grams bag (about 0.7 pounds)
- Frying oil
- Sliced spring onions – 2
- Noodles (choose from Singapore origin if you can get some) – 300 grams (0.75 pounds)

Directions

1. To prepare the bang-bang paste, mix everything in the paste ingredients part well and let it stay overnight. On the next day, take the paste and heat it in a wok or a large non-stick frying pan for 2 minutes.

2. Once it's heated, add the raw king prawns and stir-fry until they turn pink. After obtaining a pink color, remove the prawns and the paste from the wok and proceed to heat a tablespoon of oil without wiping the wok.

3. When the oil is hot, add the vegetable stir-fries and cook as you stir continuously for the next three minutes. After the third minute, add noodles and stir for another two minutes. This allows the noodles to heat through.

4. With the noodles in, put the prawns and paste back in the wok and let the food to simmer without stirring. When ready, remove the wok from heat and serve before topping every individual plate with the sliced spring onions.

36. Asparagus, Yellow Squash, and Cod

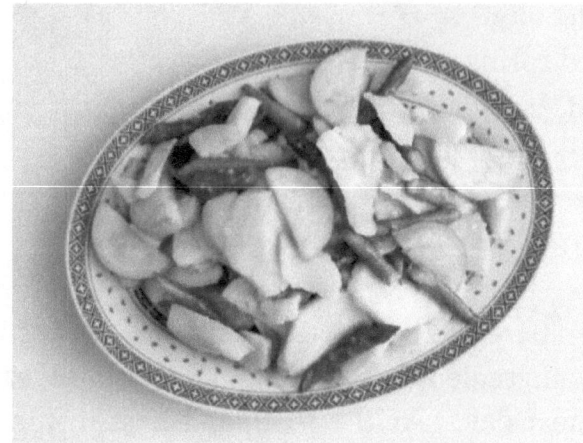

The cod is water-velveted to tenderize the meat. It is a light and delicate meal with vegetables making it a perfect dish while balancing the nutrients.

Cooking time: 45 minutes
Serving: 2

Ingredients

Cod ingredients

- Cod (or halibut – a white fish), ¼-inch slices – ½ pound
- Cornstarch – 2 teaspoons
- Lightly beaten egg white – 1 tablespoon
- Sake or Chinese rice wine- 2 teaspoons
- Kosher salt – ¼ teaspoon
- Vegetable or canola oil – 1 teaspoon

- Water – 6 cups

Stir fry ingredients

- Finely minced medium garlic clove – 1
- Low-sodium chicken stock, bought or homemade – 3 tablespoons
- Sesame oil – 1 teaspoon
- Vegetable or canola oil – 1 tablespoon
- Cornstarch – 1 teaspoon
- Yellow squash (from summer), 1/8-inch slices – ¼ pound
- Kosher salt to taste
- Garden asparagus (sparrow grass), trim ends, cut into ½-inch lengths – ¼ pound
- White rice, cooked and ready to serve

Directions

Preparing the cod

1. Take a small bowl and thoroughly mix the following: cornstarch, egg white, salt and rice wine. Put the cod in another bowl and pour the mixture you prepared in step 1 on it. Toss gently to coat the cod.

2. Once the cod is coated, refrigerate it for thirty minutes. After the sitting time, put water in a wok and bring to boil. Add oil at boiling point. After the oil, proceed to add the cod.

3. Cook and stir with a strainer or chopsticks until the outer surface is opaque but raw inside. It should take you 30 seconds.

4. When the cod becomes opaque, use a colander (bowl-shaped strainer) to remove the cod, shaking the excess water. When the wok is empty, clean the wok to dry.

Stir-fry preparation

1. Take a small bowl and mix the following: garlic, chicken stock cornstarch and sesame oil. After mixing, take the wok, this time clean and put the vegetable oil before heating until it smokes. Follow by adding asparagus and squash and proceed to cook and stir for 30 seconds.

2. Add the cod you prepared and cook as you gently stir. Continue stirring in the same manner for a minute to avoid breaking it up.

3. Once the minute is over, put sauce in the wok and season with salt. Cook and keep stirring gently until the fish and vegetables get coated and the sauce thickens. Once you get a thick sauce, remove the wok from the heat and serve with the cooked white rice.

37. Thai Green Prawn Curry

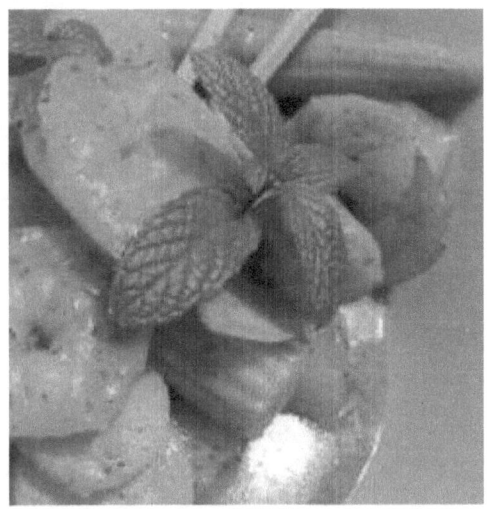

You can substitute the prawn with chicken in this recipe.

Cooking time: 35 minutes
Serving: 4

Ingredients

Paste ingredients

- Ground coriander – 1 ½ teaspoons
- Ground cumin seeds – ½ teaspoon
- Minced ginger root – 3 teaspoons
- Green chilies – 2-3
- Minced garlic cloves – 4 teaspoons
- Fresh coriander, chopped – 6 full tablespoons
- Lemongrass (or 1 ½ lemon to make lemon zest) – 3 stalks

- Lime zest – make from 1 lime
- Lime juice – squeeze 2 limes
- Frying oil – 2 tablespoons

Other ingredients

- Tiger prawns (raw or cooked), peel and remove dorsal vein – 300 grams (¾ pounds)
- Mangetout or green beans – 200 grams (½ pound)
- Frying oil – 4 tablespoons
- Coconut milk – 400ml
- Baby corn – 200 grams (½ pound)
- Soy sauce – 3 tablespoons

Directions

1. Start by doing either of the following: Put the ingredients from the paste section in a food processor to form a thick paste, smooth in nature or, chop all the ingredients (still in the same part) finely and mix thoroughly.

2. After mixing, heat a wok and then proceed to add oil. After the oil, put baby corn and beans and stir-fry for 40 seconds. Add the paste you made in step 1 together with coconut milk and let them boil lightly.

3. After the light boiling, switch the heat to medium so that the paste can simmer for 5-7 minutes.

4. After the 6th-7th minute, put the prawns in the wok then cook and stir for 3-5 minutes. If the sauce is too thick,

you can add some water. On the other hand, if it is thin, reduce the heat again.

5. After five minutes are over, remove the wok from heat and serve immediately. Best served with jasmine rice.

38. Prawn and Vegetable Omelet

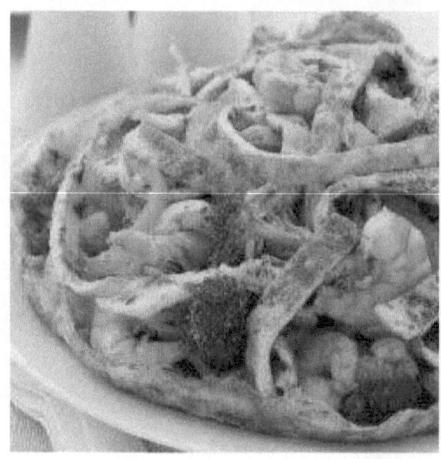

Colorful vegetables with a layer of omelet add taste to the prawn.

Cooking time: 30 minutes
Serving: 4

Ingredients

- Raw prawns, peel, thawed (unfreeze) and drained – 350 grams (0.8 pounds)
- Toasted sesame oil – 1 teaspoon
- Eggs – 8
- Fresh and chopped coriander – 3 tablespoons (optional)
- Light soy sauce – 1 tablespoon
- Corn flour – 2 teaspoons
- Sherry wine (medium or dry) – 2 tablespoons

- Broccoli florets, cut to thin slices – 300 grams (¾ pounds)
- Vegetable oil – 2 tablespoons
- Red or orange pepper, seeded and thinly sliced – 3
- Chopped garlic cloves – 2
- Fresh ginger root, peeled and cut into thin strips – 50 grams (2 teaspoons)
- Sliced spring onions – 4
- Bean sprouts (from germinating bean seeds) – 200 grams (½ pound)

Directions

1. In one bowl, beat the eggs together with sesame oil and coriander, if available and set aside. Proceed to take another bowl and mix corn flour, sherry, and soy sauce to form a smooth paste and set aside too.

2. Now, it's time to cook after the first two steps. In a large wok/ non-stick frying pan, heat half of the vegetable oil. Once the oil is heated, add pepper, broccoli, garlic, ginger and spring onions. After the addition, cook as you stir for about 5 minutes until the broccoli looks tender and bright green.

3. Next, pour the soy sauce mixture you prepared in step 2 to the wok and stir for a minute. Follow by adding prawns and cook for another 2 minutes. Follow by adding bean sprouts and slightly stir for one minute. The prawn should turn pink before going to the next step.

4. After the oink turn, transfer the prawn to a large bowl and cover to keep it warm. Is the wok empty? Wipe it using a kitchen paper. Once it's clean, pour the remaining oil and heat for a few seconds.

5. Slowly, put over half of the egg mixture and spread evenly using circular motions. Stir the egg once or twice and let it cook and settle for three minutes. After the third minute, slice out the omelet to loosen it and put the pieces in a serving dish.

6. Add the remaining egg mixture quickly and cook for 1-2 minutes until it appears just set. When the egg is ready, put it on a board and cut into ribbons.

7. Next, go back to the omelet you earlier set aside and sprinkle the vegetables with a spoon. Finally, sprinkle the omelet ribbons on top before serving.

39. Scallops and Asparagus

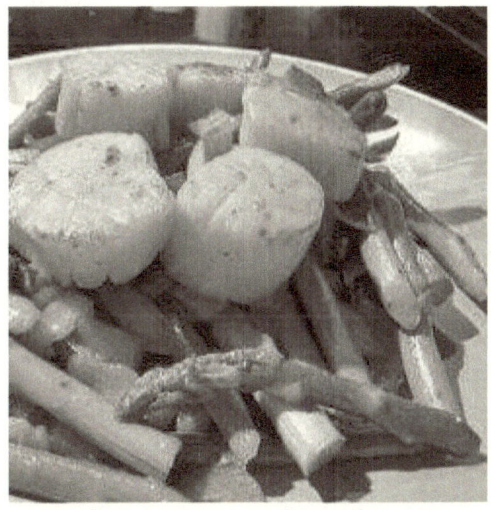

Cooking time: 30 minutes
Serving: 4

Ingredients

- Scallops, thawed (unfreeze) if frozen – 5-8 large ones
- Frying oil – 1 teaspoon and one tablespoon, separate
- Asparagus, trimmed and chopped into 3 cm pieces – 15 spears (pieces)
- Salt and pepper – as preferred
- Corn flour – as preferred
- Garlic, chopped – 1 tablespoon
- Medium onion, chopped – 1
- Finely chopped shallot – 1
- Water – 125ml (about a cup)
- Salt to taste

- Chicken stock granules (bought) – 1 teaspoon (or two teaspoons of chicken broth)
- Corn flour mixed with water – 1 teaspoon and two teaspoons respectively
- Red pepper, cut into cubes – ½
- Sesame oil – 1 teaspoon

Directions

1. Start by briefly cooking the asparagus in boiling water for three minutes together with a teaspoon of oil. After the third minute, set it aside.

2. Next, put the scallops in a bowl and season them with salt and pepper. After seasoning, cover them lightly with corn flour. After preparing the scallops, heat a tablespoon of oil over high heat.

3. When the pan is hot, put the shallot and garlic. Stir-fry them for 2-3 minutes until fragrance. At this point, add onions and salt and proceed to cook for 3-4 minutes until the onions go soft. Put the scallops and stir-fry for another 3-4 minutes until both sides have an even brown color.

4. After the scallops go brown, switch the heat to medium and add chicken stock granules (or chicken broth) then let everything to simmer for 2 minutes. Next, put red pepper in and stir. Follow by switching the heat back to high.

5. Once the heat is at high level, add the cornflour mixture, asparagus, sesame oil, and salt. Stir as the sauce heats through until it is slightly thick. When it's ready, remove the pan from heat and serve.

40. Squid with Thai Basil

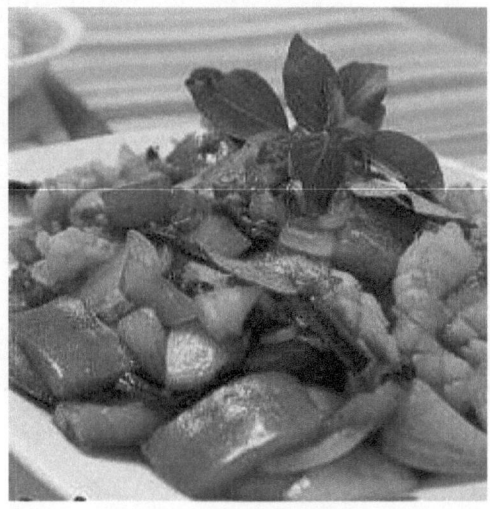

You can substitute with local basil. Serve the squid during lunch or dinner with white rice.

Cooking time: 45 minutes
Serving: 4

Ingredients

- Squid tubes, halved, mark with knife cuts (score) and cut to bite size – 2
- Corn flour – as preferred
- Salt and pepper
- Frying oil – 2 tablespoons and one tablespoon separated
- Chopped spring onions – 2
- Chopped garlic – 2 teaspoons
- Shallot, cut into dices – 1

- Salt – ½ teaspoon
- Chopped onion – 1 medium size
- Green pepper, chopped – 1
- Hot pepper sauce – 1 tablespoon
- Fish sauce – 3 tablespoons
- Water – 1 tablespoon
- Sugar – ½ teaspoon
- Thai basil leaves (or just basil leaves) – 30 grams (check in oriental stores if your local supermarket does not provide).

Directions

1. Put the squid in a bowl and season with corn flour, salt, and pepper. After seasoning, set it aside for 15 minutes. After fifteen minutes are over, take a wok or a large frying pan and heat two tablespoons of oil over high heat.

2. In the hot oil, put the squid and stir-fry for 3-5 minutes until it becomes opaque. At this point, scoop it out and set it aside. Back to the wok/frying pan, heat another tablespoon of oil over high heat.

3. When hot, sprinkle the spring onions, garlic and shallot. Stir as you let them cook for 2-3 minutes until fragrance. Follow by adding onions together with salt and lower the heat to medium. Let it cook for 3-4 minutes so that the onions can soften.

4. When the onions soften, as you stir, put the fish sauce, hot pepper sauce, green pepper, sugar, and water. Allow

everything to cook for 1-2 minutes until they are all heated through. Are they ready? If they are, remove the wok from heat and serve.

41. Cucumber and Vietnamese Seafood

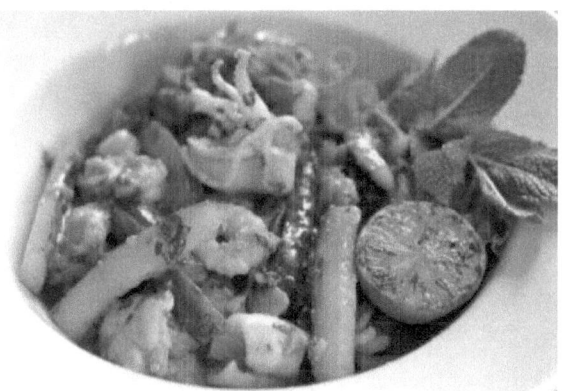

It is an impressive meal for the midweek. The cucumber blends well with shrimp sauce among other ingredients on the list.

Cooking time: 45 minutes
Serving: 4

Ingredients

- Small squid, scored (cut as if marking the flesh), cut into small pieces – 300 grams (¾ pounds)
- Tiger prawns, deveined – 300 grams (¾ pounds)
- Cucumber, slice into half, remove the seeds and cut into thin rods – 2
- Halved scallops – 4
- Large spring onions, cut white parts into rings and green parts broad diagonal slices, separate them – 2
- Finely chopped garlic cloves - 2
- Red chili, seed all, chop one to fine pieces and the other to broad pieces – 2

- Brown sugar – 2 teaspoons
- Shrimp sauce/paste – 1 tablespoon
- Halved limes – 3
- Frying oil
- Fish sauce – 1 tablespoon
- Coriander and mint, all chopped – 1 each or as preferred

Directions

1. Heat the wok over high heat. When heated, add a substantial amount of oil followed by the shrimp paste. Quickly fry for about a minute and then add the finely chopped chili, white parts of spring onions and garlic.

2. Once they are all in, cook as you stir the garlic and onions for one minute and then proceed to add the following: cucumber, fish sauce, sugar and a squeeze of one of the limes.

3. Add the seafood parts (squid and tiger prawns) and cook over the high heat for 2 minutes until they are all heated through. Is the seafood cooked through? Proceed to season with the sliced chili, half lime and green parts of the spring onions.

4. After a gentle stir, sprinkle the chopped coriander and mint and remove the wok from heat. You can also leave the cut parts (coriander and mint) on the side for the guests to season on their plates.

42. Seafood with Fried Rice

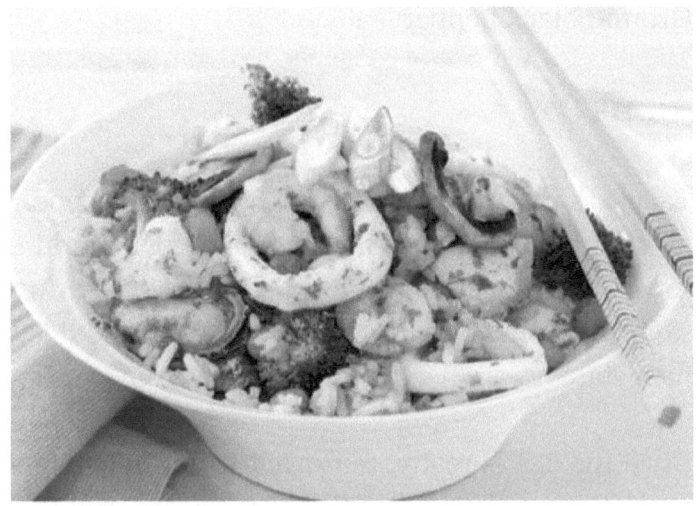

Cooking time: 25 minutes
Serving: 4

Ingredients

- White rice, cooked and ready to serve – 4 cups
- Lightly whisked egg – 1
- Onion, peel and cut into dices – 1
- Seafood marinara mix (from the store) – 500 grams
- Sliced garlic cloves – 2
- Carrot, diced into fine pieces – 1
- Broccoli, dice to small pieces – ½
- Frozen peas – 1 cup
- White mushrooms, button type, sliced – 100 grams (¼ pound)
- Soy sauce – 2 tablespoons
- Spring onions, sliced diagonally – 1

- Oyster sauce – 1 teaspoon
- Frying oil – 2 tablespoons
- Ground black pepper – 1

Directions

1. Take a small frying pan and heat a tablespoon of oil using medium heat. When the oil gets hot, add the egg as you stir in a circular motion. Continue stirring in the same motion until it appears set. You should reach a firm state before heading to the next step.

2. Once the egg is ready, remove it from the pan and let it cool off on a plate. After the heat release, roll the egg to form a cigar shape and slice it to create ribbons.

3. Now, it's time to switch to a bigger pan or a wok. Put oil in it (whatever you choose) and heat strongly. When the oil begins to simmer, immediately add the marinara mix. Start cooking as you stir for 3-4 minutes.

4. After the fourth minute, remove the mix from the wok/pan and put it aside. With the wok/pan in the same condition, put the onion and cook in a stirring manner for one minute before adding carrot and garlic.

5. Watch the garlic as it begins to color then add rice. Start tossing to mix and break any rice lumps formed in the process.

6. Once you are done tossing, add broccoli, peas, and mushrooms and go on to stir fry for the next 3-4 minutes.

7. When the mushrooms release their water, put the marinara mix back in the wok/frying pan. Add oyster and soy sauces then gently stir in the egg. Finally, season the seafood with pepper and spring onions before serving.

43. Garlic Seafood Marinara

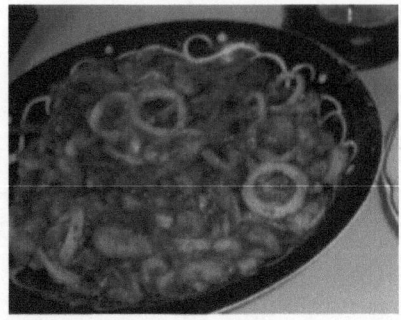

Cooking time: 40 minutes
Serving: 4

Ingredients

- Seafood marinara mix – 600 grams
- Crushed garlic cloves – 4
- Ginger, peeled, cut into matchsticks – 1
- Carrot, peeled, into matchsticks – 1
- Celery salt (from the stores) – 1 teaspoon
- Peanut oil – 3 tablespoon

Sauce ingredients

- Chicken broth – ½ cup
- Oyster sauce – 2 tablespoons
- Water – ½ cup
- Sugar – 1 tablespoon
- Corn flour – 1 tablespoon
- Soy sauce – 1 tablespoon

Directions

1. Start by thoroughly mixing the sauce ingredients and put them aside. Once the mixture is ready, heat oil in a wok until it shimmers. Proceed to add half of the crushed garlic clove and let it cook as you stir for 30 seconds.

2. After the garlic, add the seafood marinara mix. Stir-fry for 2-3 so that it is almost cooked. Is it ready? Remove the seafood mix from the wok and set it aside.

3. Without tampering with the wok, add more oil and heat vigorously. When hot, put ginger and the remaining garlic in the wok. Stir-fry them for 30 seconds to one minute.

4. After the stir, add all the vegetables (leave out spring onions). Cook and stir for about two minutes until they are slightly soft. When the veggies soften, add the marinara back to the wok followed by spring onions.

5. Now, it's time to add the sauce prepared in step 1. Stir it briefly and add to the wok. Keep cooking as you stir until the seafood is cooked through making sure you have a thick sauce. Once everything is ready, turn off the heat and serve with steamed rice.

44. Chinese Fish Fillets

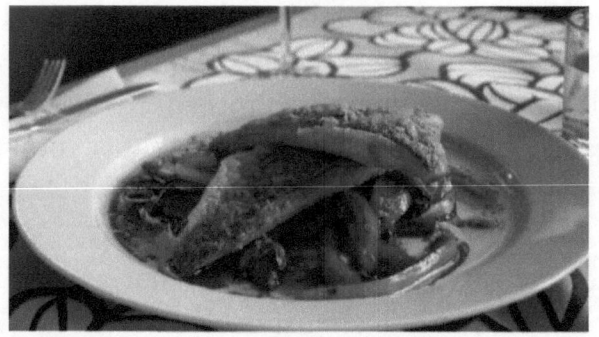

Cooking time: 25 minutes
Serving: 4

Ingredients

Fish ingredients

- Fish fillets, boneless, cut to bite size – 1 pound

Marinade ingredients

- Sesame oil – a few drops
- Sherry or white wine – 1 tablespoon
- Salt and pepper – as preferred
- Cornstarch – 2 teaspoons
- Egg white – 1 from a giant egg

Sauce ingredients

- Oyster sauce – 1 tablespoon
- Fish stock/chicken broth – ½ cup

- Cornstarch mixed with water – 1 teaspoon each
- Soy sauce – ¼ teaspoon
- Vegetable oil – 4 tablespoons
- Garlic cloves, minced – 1
- Red onion, sliced – ½
- Ginger, shredded – 2 slices
- Vegetables as desired (optional)
- Coriander, ground to taste – 2 teaspoons

Directions

Preparing the fish

1. Take a medium bowl and mix the following: sesame oil, wine, cornstarch, salt, and pepper.

2. After mixing, add fish to the mixture (marinade). Make sure it is well coated and let it sit for 10 minutes at room temperature.

Preparing the sauce

1. Take a small bowl and mix oyster and soy sauces with fish stock/chicken broth. After thorough mixing, put it aside.

2. Next, get a wok and heat two tablespoons of oil over high heat. When hot, remove the fish from the marinade, shaking off the excess and put in the wok.

3. After putting it in the wok, cook by stirring until the fish goes light brown. At this point, remove it from the wok

and put it in a bowl. With the wok in the same condition, add ginger, garlic, and red onion. Cook until the onion is light brown.

4. When the onions are ready, add the vegetables (if included) and stir-fry. After the brief stir, pour in the sauce and heat until it bubbles.

5. After the sauce looks as if it is boiling, put the cornstarch and water mixture. Stir quickly so that it thickens. After thickening, return the fish to the wok and stir everything to mix. Finally, sprinkle the ground coriander, turn off the heat and serve.

Chapter 5

Vegetables Stir-Fry Recipes

Plant-based recipes offer more nutritional value and everyone from your doctor to the next door neighbor recommends veggies for better health. So, it is the last chapter but not the least for the vegans.

Here are stir-fry recipes that will put a break on the meat.

45. Pak Choy/Bok Choy

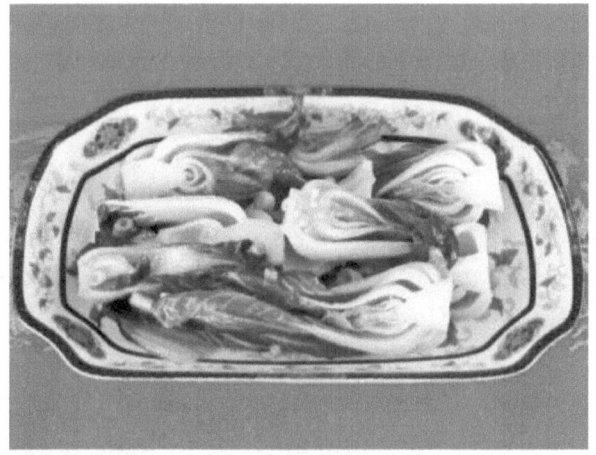

Cooking time: 10 minutes
Serving: 4

Ingredients

- Pak/bok choy, rinsed, cut the head in half lengthwise – 4 medium heads

- Ginger knob, peeled and finely sliced – 2 teaspoons
- Vegetable oil – 2 tablespoons
- Garlic cloves, peeled, and finely sliced – 2 teaspoons
- Sugar – ½ teaspoon
- Scallions, finely chopped, white parts only – 1 ½ teaspoons
- Sesame oil – 1 teaspoon
- Kosher salt

Directions

1. Start by heating the oil in a wok using medium heat until it simmers.

2. Follow by adding the following: garlic, ginger, and scallions. After the addition, cook as you stir for a minute until they are aromatic.

3. When the smell reaches you, switch the heat to high. Proceed to add the choy and stir-fry for another minute until the outer leaves wilt.

4. After wilting, add sugar, then season with salt to taste. Once the salt is in, cook and stir for one more minute.

5. At this point, it is now ready. Remove the wok from heat and add the sesame oil. Season with more salt if it's okay with you before serving.

46. Lo Mein with Charred Cabbage, Shiitake, and Chives

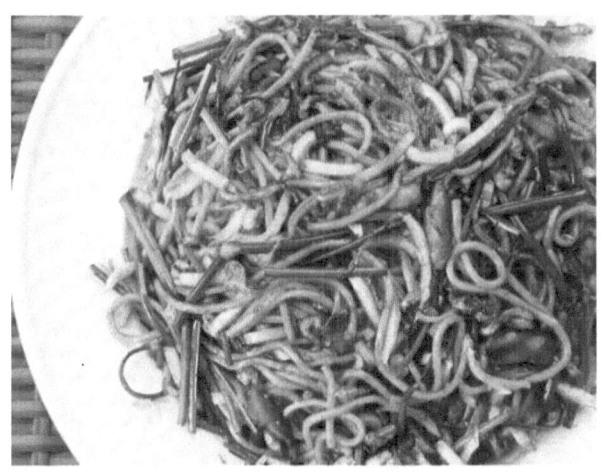

Cooking time: 30 minutes
Serving: 4

Ingredients

- Lo Mein noodles (Chinese wheat flour noodles) – 1 pound
- Kosher salt
- Vegetable or canola oil – ¼ cup, divide equally
- Shiitake mushroom caps (resemble an umbrella), thinly sliced – 4 ounces (¼ pound)
- White cabbage, shredded – 4 cups
- Fresh garlic, minced – 1 tablespoon
- Chinese chives (or scallions), cut into 2-inch segments – 4 ounces (¼ pound)
- Ground white pepper – as preferred
- Light and dark soy sauces – 2 teaspoons each

- Roasted sesame oil – 1 tablespoon
- Shaoxing wine – 1 tablespoon

Directions

1. First, boil some salted water in a pot and then add the noodles. With the noodles in the pot, stir regularly with chopsticks or tongs for a minute, until they attain a firm state but separated.

2. When ready, drain the noodles and transfer them to a large bowl. Add a tablespoon of veggie oil to the noodle's bowl and toss before setting aside.

3. Now, it's time for the wok. Take it and heat a tablespoon of oil over high heat until it smokes. Add cabbage and then cook and stir regularly for 2 minutes until they are lightly brown in color.

4. At this point, the cabbages are ready to transfer to a bowl and setting aside. You don't have to clean the wok but do so if some of the cabbage chippings are still sticking around. Now, in the empty wok, put one tablespoon of oil and heat to smoke.

5. In the hot oil, add mushrooms and proceed to cook and stir for 2 minutes or so until they brown and are somehow crisp but tender. Join the mushrooms with the chives/scallions in a stirring manner for a minute until they lightly wilt. At wilting point, transfer them to the bowl containing cabbage.

6. Clean out the wok and then heat it before adding one more tablespoon of oil and wait until it smokes. Add the noodles and toss until they become hot.

7. Once the noodles are heated, add the cabbage, chives, mushrooms, and garlic. Toss them together with noodles for 30 seconds or until you smell the garlic.

8. After the 30-second toss, put the soy sauces, sesame oil, and wine. Cook as you toss and stir until the sauce coats the noodles. Finally, season with salt and white pepper before turning off the heat. Serve while it's still hot.

47. Smacked Cucumber

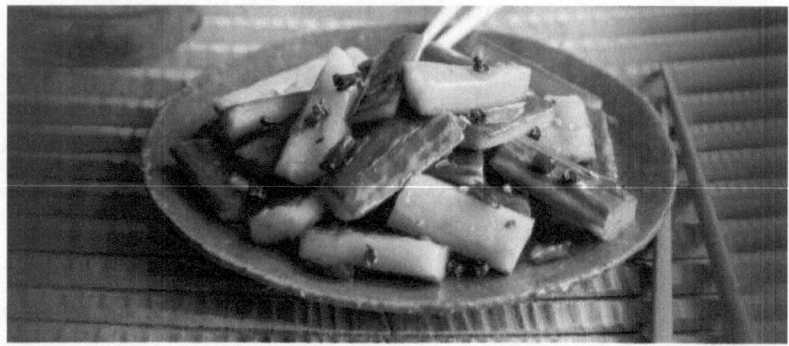

Cooking time: 50 minutes
Serving: 6

NB: You can serve it as a snack with drinks

Ingredients

- Frying oil
- Cucumber, cut into 4cm length, then chunk into wedges – 1
- Szechuan pepper – ½ teaspoon
- Red chili, dried and broken into pieces – 2
- Sesame oil

Directions

1. Take the cucumber pieces, one by one and smack them down using a cleaver's flat. Use your hands to do it. After crashing, remove the seeds and put the pieces in a sieve. Sprinkle a little salt to taste.

2. Let them settle for 30 minutes before rinsing and patting dry with paper towels. When the cucumbers are ready, heat some oil in a wok to smoking hot. In the hot oil, add chili and pepper. Follow by putting the smacked cucumber and stir for a minute.

3. After the minute, scoop the contents and put them on a plate. Remember to switch off the heat and remove the wok. Finally, sprinkle with sesame oil and serve.

48. Hoisin-Glazed Tofu (Bean Curd) and Brown Rice

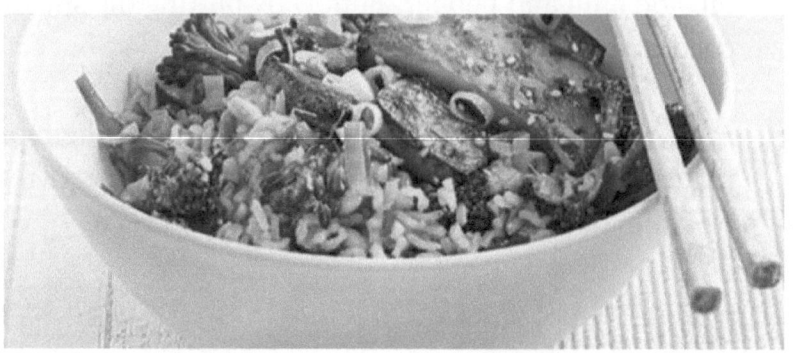

Cooking time: 30 minutes plus an hour of pressing
Serving: 2

Ingredients

- Hoisin sauce – 4 tablespoons
- Firm tofu (bean curd) – 400 grams (1 pound)
- Sesame seeds – 2 teaspoons
- Crushed garlic cloves – 2
- Grated ginger – 2 teaspoons
- Sesame oil
- Red chili, seeded, cut into dices – 1
- Spring onions, finely sliced – 1 bunch
- Brown rice, cooked – 250 grams
- Soya beans – 50 grams
- Broccoli, briefly cooked and chopped – 200 grams (½ pound)
- Soy sauce – 1 tablespoon

Directions

1. Start by cutting the tofu into strips (wide ones are preferred) and put them between two kitchen towel sheets.

2. Now you have a sandwiched tofu. Press the cut strips down using a chopping board to release some water. After the hard press, it's now ready for the next step.

3. In this step, you need the grill. Put a baking sheet with oil on it and heat it strongly before pouring the pressed tofu by brushing together with half of the hoisin.

4. Once they are all on the baking sheet, season on top with a teaspoon of sesame seeds and then grill the contents for 6-8 minutes until they turn crisp and golden.

5. Now, turn the tofu coat and add more hoisin. It's okay if you feel like scattering some more sesame seeds. Cook over the grill until you get a fragile nature before setting the tofu aside in a bowl.

6. In another setting, fry the garlic, ginger, and chili using a teaspoon of sesame oil in a wok until aromatic.

7. Next, add spring onions to the wok and stir-fry for one minute. After the onions soften, add rice and fry it for five minutes to heat through.

8. After the fifth minute, add soya and broccoli followed by soy sauce seasoning. Put the contents in bowls and top with tofu. Scatter the remaining spring onions on top and serve.

49. Aubergine (Eggplant) and Sesame Seeds

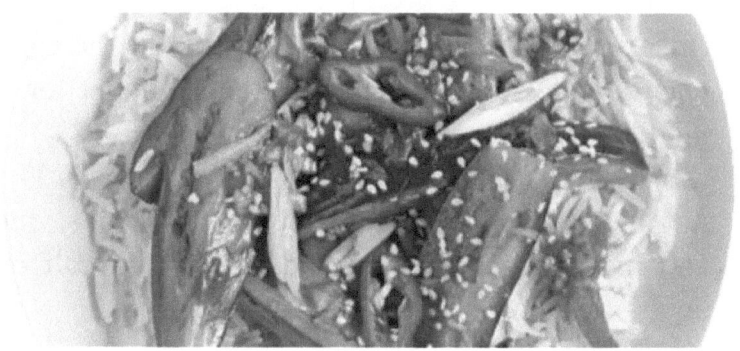

Cooking time: 30 minutes
Serving: 2

Ingredients

- Aubergines/eggplant, cut into wedges – 2 small ones
- Sliced spring onions – 2
- Sesame oil
- Crushed garlic cloves – 3
- Ginger, shredded – thumb size
- Soy sauce – 1 tablespoon
- Mirin – 1 tablespoon
- Rice wine vinegar or dry sherry – 1 tablespoon
- Sesame seeds – 1 teaspoon
- Corn flour – 1 teaspoon

Directions

1. Take a wok and heat a tablespoon of oil. When hot, stir in ginger, garlic, chili and almost all spring onions for two minutes or until aromatic.

2. Once you reach the fragrance stage, add the eggplant together with water splash. Let them simmer for 10-15 minutes to soften.

3. Add more heat and follow by putting soy sauce, vinegar, and mirin. After the addition, cook until half of the liquid is evaporated.

4. As evaporation progresses, take a bowl and mix corn flour with water splash. When you get an even mixture, stir it in the wok for two more minutes.

5. After the stir, scatter the remaining spring onions, sesame seeds, and chili slices. At this point, it is ready to serve with rice.

50. Stir-Fry Vegetables

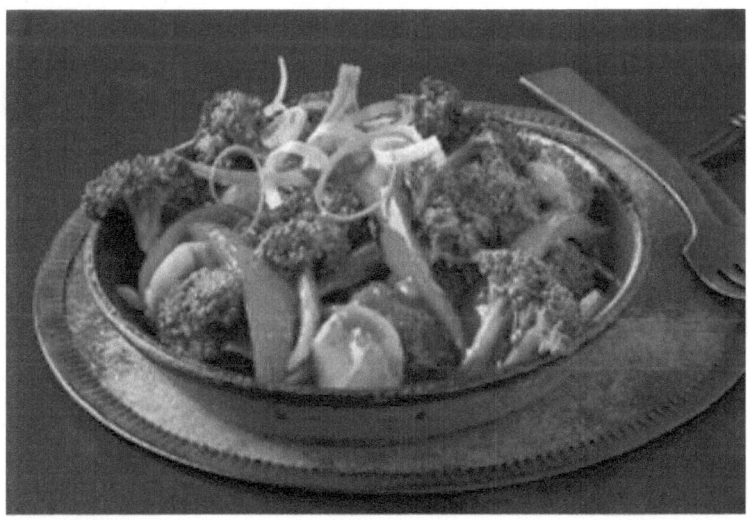

Cooking time: 20 minutes
Serving: 4

Ingredients

- Broccoli florets – 3 cups
- PLANTERS peanut oil (check the store) – 2 tablespoons
- Red pepper, cut into strips – 1 cup
- Water chestnuts (also known as Chinese water chestnuts), drained and sliced – 1 can
- Green onions, cut into slices – 3
- A.1. original sauce (produced by Kraft Foods since 1831) – 3 tablespoons
- Lemon juice – 1 teaspoon
- Soy sauce – 1 tablespoon
- Frying oil

Directions

1. Take a wok and heat a substantial amount of oil over medium to high heat. Wait for the oil to get hot before putting broccoli, onions, and pepper. Once they are all in, cook and stir for 8 minutes until the ingredients are crisp but tender.

2. After the eighth minute, put as you stir all the remaining ingredients and cook for 3-5 minutes. At this point, they are heated through. Don't stop stirring during this period. Are they ready? Turn off the heat and serve.

51. Sesame Vegetables with Rice

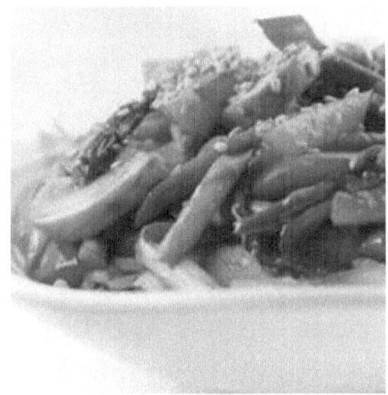

Cooking time: 35 minutes
Serving: 3

Ingredients

- Long-grain rice, uncooked – ¾ cup
- Vegetable broth – 1 ½ cups
- Fresh asparagus, trim and cut into 1-inch pieces – ½ pound
- Sesame seeds – 1 tablespoon
- Margarine – 1 tablespoon
- Peanut oil – 2 tablespoons (preferred but you can use vegetable oil, same amount)
- Large red bell pepper, cut into 1-inch pieces – 1
- Mushrooms, sliced – 2 cups
- Yellow onion, sliced – 1, large one
- Fresh and minced ginger root – 2 teaspoons
- Soy sauce – 3 tablespoons
- Minced garlic – 1 teaspoon

- Sesame oil – 1 tablespoon

Directions

1. First, you need the oven. Heat it to 175 degrees Celsius (350 degrees F). Next, take a saucepan and combine rice with broth and margarine. Cover them and heat in the oven until they boil.

2. At boiling point, reduce the heat so that the rice simmers for 15 minutes. Set the rice aside when all the liquid is absorbed.

3. Now, it's time to prepare the sesame seeds. Put them on a baking sheet and heat in the preheated oven for 5-6 minutes so that they turn golden brown. After attaining a golden color, put them aside in a separate bowl or plate.

4. With the seeds ready, head for the wok or skillet. Take it and heat the peanut oil using the medium to high heat.

5. In the hot oil, add asparagus, onion, bell pepper, ginger, mushrooms, and garlic. Proceed to stir-fry them for 4-5 minutes until the veggies become tender but still crisp. The above inputs are followed by stirring in the soy sauce and let it cook for 30 seconds.

6. After the sauce, turn off the heat. While it's still hot, put toasted sesame seeds and sesame oil and stir before serving over the rice.

52. Garbanzo

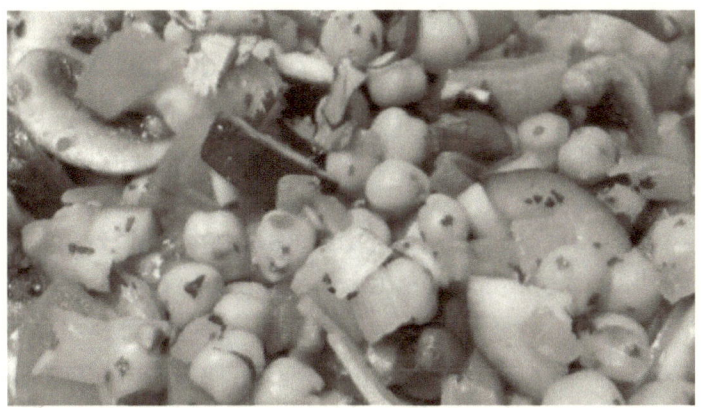

Cooking time: 35 minutes
Serving: 3

Ingredients

- Rinsed and drained Garbanzo beans – 1 can
- Fresh oregano (of the mint family), chopped – 1 tablespoon
- Olive oil – 2 tablespoons
- Fresh and chopped basil – 1 tablespoon
- Black pepper, ground – as preferred
- Crushed garlic cloves – 1
- Large zucchini, half and slice it – 1
- Fresh coriander or cilantro (same family), chopped – 1 tablespoon
- Sliced mushrooms – ½ cup
- Chopped tomato – 1

Directions

1. Take a large skillet/wok and heat oil using medium heat. In the hot oil, put oregano, garlic, basil, and pepper and keep stirring as you put each of the ingredients.

2. After stirring all the ingredients, add zucchini and garbanzo beans and stir everything to coat.

3. Next, cover the food and let it cook but keep stirring once in a while. It should take you 10 minutes.

4. When ten minutes are over, put the cilantro/coriander and mushrooms in a stirring motion. Continue to stir as the mixture cooks until they reach a tender state. When the mushrooms tenderize, place the tomato on the mixture and don't mix.

5. Cover the food and let the tomato steam for some minutes. Don't allow it to get mushy. When the food is ready, turn off the heat and serve while it's still hot.

53. Broccoli Noodles and Spicy Mushroom

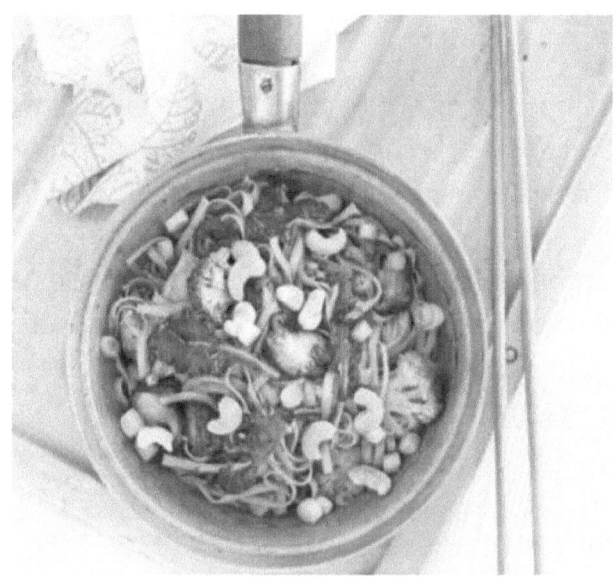

Cooking time: 20 minutes
Serving: 2

Ingredients

- Vegetable stock cube, with low-salt – 1
- Small head broccoli florets – 1
- Medium egg noodles – 2 nests (about 125 grams)
- Shiitake/chestnut mushroom, cut into thick slices – 250 grams
- Sesame oil – 1 tablespoon, preserve more for serving
- Large garlic clove, chopped – 1
- Thinly sliced spring onions – 4
- Dried chili, break down into pieces – ½ teaspoon

- Hoisin sauce – 2 tablespoons
- Roasted cashew nuts – a handful

Directions

1. Start by putting water in a pan and boil the vegetable stock cube. At boiling point, add egg noodles and then let them simmer together for 2 minutes.

2. After the second minute, put broccoli in the pan and let it boil for another two minutes. When ready, turn off the heat and reserve a cup of the 'stock broth' before draining the rest.

3. Next, heat a wok/large non-stick frying pan and add sesame oil and mushrooms. Stir-fry them for two minutes until they turn golden.

4. After the mushrooms stir, add chili flakes, garlic, and almost all spring onions. Cook them for a minute before adding the boiled broccoli and noodles.

5. Once the noodles and broccoli are in, splash three tablespoons of the reserved stock. Follow by putting hoisin sauce and toss for another minute using two wooden spoons or a pair of tongs.

6. When everything is ready, turn off the heat and serve the noodles sprinkled with the toasted cashew nuts and the rest of spring onions. If it's okay, you can add some sesame oil for the taste.

54. Seitan (Wheat Gluten) and Black Bean

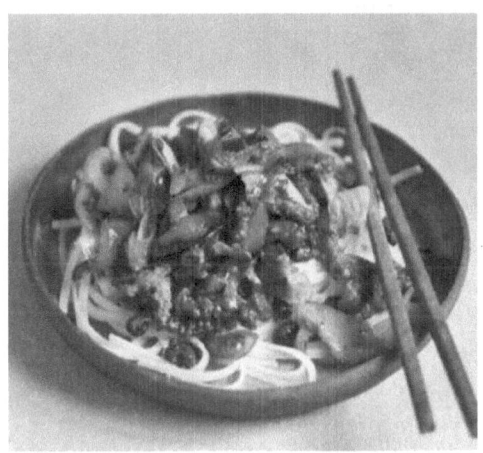

Cooking time: 45 minutes
Serving: 4

Ingredients

Sauce ingredients

- Dark brown sugar, soft granules – 75 grams (about 0.2 pounds)
- Rinsed and drained black beans – 400 grams
- Garlic cloves – 3
- Chinese five-spice (check the stores) – 1 teaspoon
- Soy sauce – 2 tablespoons
- Rice vinegar – 2 tablespoons
- Red chili, chop into fine pieces – 1
- Smooth peanut butter – 1 tablespoon

Stir-fry ingredients

- Corn flour – 1 tablespoon
- Marinated seitan (wheat gluten) pieces – 350 grams
- Sliced red pepper – 1
- Vegetable oil – 3 tablespoons
- Chopped pak choi – 300 grams (¾ pounds)
- Sliced spring onions – 2
- Rice or rice noodles, cooked and ready to serve.

Directions

1. In the food processor bowl, prepare the sauce by putting beans and ingredients in the sauce section. Add 50ml of water and blend to a smooth texture.

2. When blended, pour the sauce into a saucepan and gently heat for five minutes until thick and shiny before setting it aside in a bowl.

3. Next, drain the seitan and dry with paper towels. Put the pieces in a bowl with corn flour and toss before setting the coated seitan pieces aside.

4. After the coating exercise, heat a wok over high heat then add some oil and seitan in batches.

5. Cook and stir them for 5 minutes until the edges turn golden brown. After the color turn, use a slotted spoon to remove the seitan from the wok and put aside in a plate.

6. Now, dry the empty wok and add a teaspoon of vegetable oil. Wait for the oil to heat before putting all the beans, pepper, spring onions and pak choi. Once they are all in, cook them in a stirring manner for 3-4 minutes.

7. After the fourth minute, return the seitan and stir to coat with the sauce before letting it boil for a minute. Finally, when everything is ready, switch off the heat and serve together with rice or noodles.

55. Gingered Tofu, Pea Noodles and Aubergine (Eggplant)

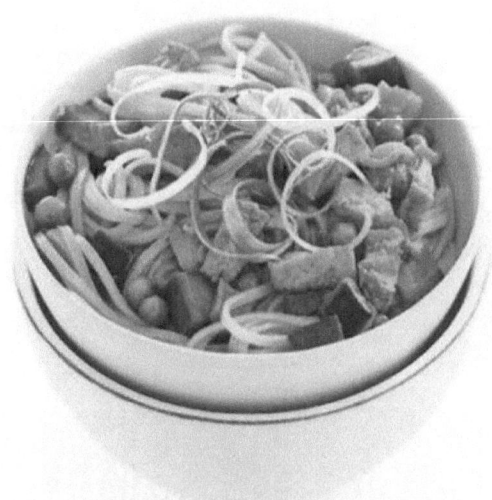

Cooking time: 25 minutes
Serving: 4

Ingredients

- Aubergines/eggplant, cut into small chunks – 2
- Toasted sesame oil – 3 tablespoons
- Garlic cloves – 1
- Medium egg noodles – 4 nests (about 250 grams)
- Grated ginger – thumb size
- Soy sauce – 3 tablespoons
- Chinese five-spice powder – 2 teaspoons (from the stores or check on how to make one)
- Marinated tofu (bean curd) pieces – 160 grams (0.4 pounds)

- Sweet chili sauce – 3 tablespoons
- Spring onions, shred – 3
- Frozen peas (unfrozen) – 225 grams (about ½ pound)

Directions

1. First, cook the noodles according to package instructions. When the noodles are ready, take a wok, or a large non-stick frying pan and heat over high heat then add two tablespoons of oil.

2. In the hot oil, put the aubergine/eggplant pieces and proceed to cook and stir them for 8-10 minutes until they turn brown and completely soft. At this point, remove the eggplant pieces from the wok/frying pan and add the remaining tablespoon of oil.

3. Wait for the oil to get hot before putting ginger and garlic. Let them cook for 30 seconds without stirring. Then, as you stir, put the five-spice.

4. Next, with the help of a spoon, put the chili and soy sauces then stir as you let it bubble for another 30 seconds. After the bubble, toss in the tofu, eggplant pieces, and peas. Cook as you stir until they are all heated through.

5. Before you serve, add the noodles and toss to mix everything. Finally, turn off the heat and serve in the respective bowls. Let the guests season with spring onions on their plates as desired.

Conclusion

By now, you are familiar with recipes that will arm your kitchen with ingredients and instructions on how to use them as you look forward to achieve the best results of each recipe. Most of them will be switched from one recipe to another so if you note something that you'll be using often, buy it in bulk.

It is actually recommendable that after reading this book, purchase what is common in the methods you pick in large quantities.

Stir-frying cuisine can be hard to grasp especially when searching for the actual ingredients so, you are allowed to substitute when necessary. It will affect the overall texture and taste, but that does not mean you are ruining everything. Regardless of the substitution, all ingredients must be attended to as instructed.

One more thing, you only need one primary cooking instrument, a wok – the definition of stir-frying art. Other named equipment is also valid. So, depending on the quantity, choose something that will fit everything and won't get in the way of stir-frying as you cook.

Having captured what you need for a quick stir-fry recipe, what remains is for you to try and see what awaits you on the other end.

All the best as you stir-fry!

Final Words

I would like to thank you for purchasing my book and I hope I have been able to help you and educate you on something new.

If you have enjoyed this book and would like to share your positive thoughts, could you please take 30 seconds of your time to go back and give me a review on my Amazon book page.

I greatly appreciate seeing these reviews because it helps me share my hard work.

You can leave me a review on Amazon.com.

Again, thank you and I wish you all the best!

www.ingramcontent.com/pod-product-compliance
Lightning Source LLC
Chambersburg PA
CBHW031115080526
44587CB00011B/984